NANDA List of Nursing Diagnoses
Organized According to Gordon's Functional Health Patterns

Health Perception-Health Management Pattern
Aspiration, Potential For*
Denial, Ineffective
Health Maintenance, Altered
Health Seeking Behavior (Specify)*
Infection, Potential For
Injury, Potential For
Noncompliance
Poisoning, Potential For
Suffocation, Potential For
Trauma, Potential For

Nutritional-Metabolic Pattern
Breastfeeding, Ineffective*
Body Temperature, Potential Altered
Dysreflexia*
Fluid Volume Deficit, Actual
Fluid Volume Deficit, Potential
Fluid Volume Excess
Nutrition, Altered: Less Than Body Requirements
Nutrition, Altered: More Than Body Requirements
Nutrition, Altered: Potential For More Than Body Requirements
Hyperthermia
Hypothermia†
Skin Integrity, Impaired
Skin Integrity, Potential Impaired
Thermoregulation, Ineffective
Tissue Integrity, Impaired
Swallowing, Impaired
Oral Mucous Membrane, Altered‡

Elimination
Bowel Incontinence‡
Constipation‡
Constipation, Colonic*
Constipation, Perceived*
Diarrhea‡
Urinary Elimination, Altered Patterns of
(Urinary) Incontinence: Functional
(Urinary) Incontinence: Reflex
(Urinary) Incontinence: Stress
(Urinary) Incontinence: Total
(Urinary) Incontinence: Urge
Urinary Retention

Activity-Exercise Pattern
Activity Intolerance
Activity Intolerance, Potential
Airway Clearance, Ineffective
Breathing Pattern, Ineffective
Cardiac Output, Decreased‡
Disuse, Potential For*
Diversional Activity Deficit
Fatigue
Growth and Development, Altered
Gas Exchange, Impaired
Home Maintenance Management, Impaired
Mobility, Impaired Physical
Self-Care Deficit, Bathing/Hygiene*‡
Self-Care Deficit, Dressing/Grooming‡
Self-Care Deficit, Feeding‡
Self-Care Deficit, Toileting‡
Tissue Perfusion, Altered (Specify): Renal, Cerebral, Cardiopulmonary, Gastrointestinal, Peripheral‡

Sleep-Rest Pattern
Sleep Pattern Disturbance

Cognitive-Perceptual Pattern
Conflict, Decisional (Specify)*
Knowledge Deficit (Specify)
Pain‡
Pain, Chronic
Sensory/Perceptual Alterations: Visual, Auditory, Kinesthetic, Gustatory, Tactile, Olfactory
Thought Processes, Altered
Unilateral Neglect

Self-Perception/Self-Concept Pattern
Anxiety
Body Image Disturbance‡
Fear
Hopelessness
Personal Identify Disturbance‡
Powerlessness
Self-Esteem Disturbance†‡
Self-Esteem Disturbance, Situational Low*
Self-Esteem Disturbance, Chronic Low*

Role-Relationship Pattern
Conflict, Parental Role*
Communication, Impaired Verbal§
Coping, Defensive*
Family Processes, Altered
Grieving, Anticipatory
Grieving, Dysfunctional‖
Parenting, Altered
Parenting, Potential Altered
Role Performance, Altered‡
Social Interaction, Impaired
Social Isolation
Violence, Potential For

Sexuality-Reproductive Pattern
Sexuality, Altered Patterns
Sexual Dysfunction
Rape-Trauma Syndrome
Rape-Trauma Syndrome: Compound Reaction
Rape-Traume Syndrome: Silent Reaction

Coping-Stress Pattern
Adjustment, Impaired
Coping, Family: Potential For Growth
Coping, Ineffective Family: Compromised
Coping, Ineffective Family: Disabled
Coping, Ineffective Individual
Post-Trauma Response

Value-Belief Pattern
Spiritual Distress

---

*New diagnostic category approved 1988
†Revised diagnostic category approved 1988
‡Category label name modified 1988

§Author recommends adding Impaired Communication (if you can't understand words, then you won't be able to respond appropriately verbally).
‖Author recommends adding Grieving (normal) to the list.

Applying Nursing Diagnosis and Nursing Process:

A Step-by-Step Guide

SECOND EDITION

Rosalinda Alfaro, RN, MSN

Lecturer, Nursing Division
Immaculata College
Immaculata, Pennsylvania

Co-adjunct Instructor
Nursing Division
Delaware County Community College
Media, Pennsylvania

Staff Nurse (per diem)
Intensive Care Units
Paoli Memorial Hospital
Paoli, Pennsylvania

J.B. Lippincott Company   Philadelphia

Grand Rapids   New York   St. Louis   San Francisco
London   Sydney   Tokyo

Acquisitions Editor: Patricia L. Cleary
Developmental Editor: Rosanne Hallowell
Project Editor: Lynda Kenny
Indexer: Sandra King
Design Director: Susan Hess Blaker
Design Coordinator: Doug Smock
Production Manager: Carol A. Florence
Production Coordinator: Pamela Milcos
Compositor: Circle Graphics
Text Printer/Binder: R. R. Donnelley & Sons Company, Inc.
Cover Printer: Phoenix

   3   5   6   4

Library of Congress Cataloging-in-Publication Data

Alfaro, Rosalinda.
  Applying nursing diagnosis and nursing process.

  Rev. ed. of: Application of nursing process. c1986.
  Includes bibliographies and index.
  1. Nursing—Handbooks, manuals, etc. 2. Diagnosis—
Handbooks, manuals, etc. I. Alfaro, Rosalinda.
Application of nursing process. II. Title.
[DNLM: 1. Nursing Process—methods. WY 100 A385a]
RT51.A6Z55 1990   610.73   88-27207
ISBN 0-397-54769-2

Any procedure or practice described in this book should be applied by the healthcare practitioner under appropriate supervision in accordance with professional standards of care used with regard to the unique circumstances that apply in each practice situation. Care has been taken to confirm the accuracy of information presented and to describe generally accepted practices. However, the authors, editors, and publisher cannot accept any responsibility for errors or omissions or for consequences from application of the information in this book and make no warranty, express or implied, with respect to the contents of the book.

Every effort has been made to ensure drug selections, and dosages are in accordance with current recommendations and practice. Because of ongoing research, changes in government regulations and the constant flow of information on drug therapy, reactions, and interactions, the reader is cautioned to check the package insert for each drug for indications, dosages, warnings, and precautions, particularly if the drug is new or infrequently used.

For my parents, Margaret and Jimmy.

And for Dianne, Tuck, Michael, Jim, Matt,
Janet, Dennis, Daniel, Chelsey, Chuck, Chris, Anne Marie,
Ledjie, Heidi, Craig, Eric, Ellie, Holly, and Becky.

Consultants

My gratitude goes to the consultants listed below. Their time, suggestions, and critiques were invaluable in pulling this project together.

Ledjie Ballard, RN, MSN, CRNA
Chief Nurse Anesthetist
Group Health Cooperative
East Side Hospital
Seattle, Washington

Lynda Carpenito, RN, MSN
LJC Consultants
Mickleton, New Jersey

Nancy Chiarantona, RN, MSN
Assistant Professor
Nursing Division
Gwynedd Mercy College
Gwynedd Valley, Pennsylvania

Nancy Flynn, RN, MSN
Clinical Educator
Medical-Surgical
Bryn Mawr Hospital
Bryn Mawr, Pennsylvania

Terri Patterson, RN, MSN, CRRN
Nursing Consultation Services,
 Ltd.
2497 Fieldcrest Ave.
Norristown, Pennsylvania

Rebecca Resh, M.Ed.
Mediplex Rehab—Camden
Director, Cognitive Remediation/
 Special Educ.
Camden, New Jersey

Constance Sechrist, RN
Staff Nurse
Hospital of the University of
 Pennsylvania
Philadelphia, Pennsylvania

Mary Carol Taylor, CSFN, RN, MSN
Division of Nursing
Holy Family College
Philadelphia, Pennsylvania

Diane Verity, B.S.
Biopharmaceutical Production
 R & D
Centocor, Inc.
Malvern, Pennsylvania

Preface

As with the previous edition,* this second edition of *Applying Nursing Diagnosis and Nursing Process: A Step-by-Step Guide* has been written with the intent of providing a text which combines the *theory* and the *real world* of nursing process. For each activity, I have sought to provide the answer to the following questions:

Why, *in theory,* are nurses required to use the nursing process?
How, *in reality,* are nurses *using* the nursing process?
How can we help nurses to use the nursing process in the *safest, most efficient, and most effective way?*

Based upon comments and suggestions on the first edition from educators, students, and practicing nurses, much of this book has been rewritten to incorporate new ideas and material. Most specifically you will find the following:

☐ More information on the collaborative role of the nurse. Every effort has been made to give a balance of information on both the *independent role* and the *interdependent, or collaborative, role* of the nurse. (Nurses need to be able to apply the nursing process to *both* roles.)

☐ More information on the process of making a diagnosis (use of *diagnostic reasoning*). This includes principles, steps, and rules that can be used as guides or reviews for using both logic and intuition to make a diagnosis.

☐ A *Nursing Diagnosis Quick Reference* section that provides quick retrieval of definitions, defining characteristics, and contributing/relating factors for each of the diagnoses accepted for study and testing by the North American Nursing Diagnosis Association (NANDA).

---

*This edition has been retitled (the previous edition was entitled *Application of Nursing Process: A Step-by-Step Guide*) to reflect the greater emphasis on nursing diagnosis. Chapter 3 has been significantly expanded, and a Quick Reference to Nursing Diagnoses section has been added.

☐ A greater emphasis on the identification and utilization of *client strengths*.

☐ Principles and steps for setting priorities during both the planning and implementation phases of the nursing process.

☐ More information on the role of goals as key factors in planning and evaluating nursing care.

☐ More practice sessions to reinforce key points and to encourage active participation on the part of the reader.

By presenting this information in a step-by-step format, with a strong emphasis on the rationale for every activity, it is my hope that students, educators, and practitioners will have a resource that really meets their needs, both in theory and in practice.

Whenever possible, I have used a fictitious person's name in place of "the client" or "the patient" to help us to keep in mind that each client or patient is an individual who has unique needs, beliefs, values, perceptions, and motivations.

Keeping in mind that students and nurses have to do a lot of reading in a short period of time, I have worked very hard to provide a text that is comprehensive, concise, interesting, and fun. I welcome and appreciate comments for improvement, and request that any suggestions be directed to me, in care of the J. B. Lippincott Company or Immaculata College.

Rosalinda Alfaro RN, MSN

Acknowledgments

I want to thank Nat and Louise Rochester for getting me started on the computer, and for working vacations in Duxbury, Massachusetts.

Also, the following people for their belief in me, and for their contribution to my personal and professional growth: John Payne, Charlie Lindsay, Patti Cleary, Mary Jo Boyer, Lynda Carpenito, Heidi Laird, Ledjie Ballard, Diane Verity, Debbie Sowers, Annette Sophocles, Becky Resh, Jim LeFevre, Nancy Flynn, Carol Taylor, Lois Blatman, Lynda Kenny, Karen Braithwaite, the faculties of Villanova University School of Nursing and Immaculata College, and the present and past staff nurses of Paoli Memorial Hospital.

Contents

Applying
Nursing Diagnosis and
Nursing Process:

A Step-by-Step Guide

SECOND EDITION

Introduction

This book is intended to help make the nursing process make sense to you. I have purposely made the reading as easy as possible and have used many real-life examples and situations to make learning this material both interesting and relevant. I have also incorporated real-life situations into practice sessions that are specifically designed to give you the opportunity to become actively involved in using the steps of the nursing process.

It is my hope that you will use this book in whatever way you find most helpful; for example, if you need added clarification, write it on the pages. Mark it up and make it yours. Do the practice sessions when you feel you need clarification. Omit them if you feel that you already understand the content. The answers to the practice sessions are in the back of the book for your referral, but try to do the sessions on your own before checking the answers. These practice sessions are for *your* benefit, and you should use them in whatever way you find most helpful.

The ANA standards for nursing practice (listed below) provide the foundation for the nursing process as described in this book.

American Nurses' Association Standards for Practice

I. The collection of data about the health status of the client/patient is systematic and continuous. The data are accessible, communicated, and recorded.

II. Nursing diagnoses are derived from health status data.

III. The plan of nursing care includes goals derived from the nursing diagnoses.

IV. The plan of nursing care includes priorities and the prescribed nursing approaches or measures to achieve the goals derived from the nursing diagnoses.

V. Nursing actions provide for client/patient participation in health promotion, maintenance, and restoration.

VI. Nursing actions assist the client/patient to maximize his health capabilities.

VII. The client's/patient's progress or lack of progress toward goal achievement is determined by the client/patient and the nurse.

VIII. The client's/patient's progress or lack of progress toward goal achievement directs reassessment, reordering of priorities, new goal setting, and revision of the plan of nursing care.

*Abstracted from Standards of Nursing Practice. Copyright © American Nurses' Association, 1973.

☑ Assessment
☑ Diagnosis
☑ Planning
☑ Implementation
☑ Evaluation

1 Nursing Process Overview

Glossary

Analyze To examine and categorize pieces of information to determine where they might fit into the "whole picture."

Assessment The first step of the nursing process, during which data are gathered and examined in preparation for the second step, diagnosis.

Diagnosis The second step of the nursing process, during which data are analyzed and pulled together for the purpose of identifying and describing health status (strengths, and actual and potential health problems).

Evaluation The fifth step of the nursing process, during which the extent of goal achievement is determined; each of the previous four steps is analyzed to identify factors that enhanced or hindered progress, and the plan of care is modified or terminated as indicated.

Implementation The fourth step of the nursing process, which involves putting the plan of care into action.

Nursing Intervention An action performed by a nurse to prevent illness (or its complications) and to promote, maintain, or restore health, or to assist a patient with a terminal condition to achieve a peaceful death.

Nursing Process An organized, systematic method of giving individualized nursing care that focuses on identifying and treating unique responses of individuals or groups to actual or potential alterations in health.

Medical Treatment Plan The plan used by physicians to treat diseases (focuses upon correcting pathology or injury to organs or systems).

Planning The third step of the nursing process, during which goals are set, interventions are identified, and a plan of nursing care is developed.

Synthesize To bring together pieces of information to give a clear picture of the whole.

What Is the Nursing Process?

In the following chapters, you will be able to study each step of the nursing process in depth. But for now, let's take a broad look at what the nursing process means. What is it? How does it work? Why should we use it?

Basically, the nursing process is an organized, systematic method of giving individualized nursing care that focuses upon identifying and treating unique responses of individuals or groups to actual or potential alterations in health. It consists of five steps—assessment, diagnosis, planning, implementation, and evaluation—during which the nurse performs deliberate activities to achieve the ultimate goals of nursing:

☐ To promote, maintain or restore health, or to assist patients to achieve a peaceful death, when their condition is terminal

☐ To enable individuals or groups to manage their own healthcare to the best of their ability

☐ To provide nursing care that is of the best quality and efficiency possible

Here is a brief description of the types of activities that you will be doing during each step of the nursing process.

Steps of the Nursing Process

☐ **Assessment:** During the assessment phase, you will need to gather and examine information (data) to obtain all the facts necessary to determine your patient's health status and to describe strengths and problems.

☐ **Diagnosis:** Once you have all the necessary facts, you will be ready to analyze the data to identify *strengths* (which will be reinforced and used in developing the plan of care) and *actual and potential problems* (which will be the basis for the plan of care). You will also determine which problems can be resolved through independent nursing interventions, and which problems will require interventions that must be prescribed by a physician or other qualified healthcare professional.

☐ **Planning:** Once you have identified strengths and problems, you are ready to work with your patient (and family) to *develop a plan of action* that will reduce or eliminate the problems and promote health. Planning includes the following key activities:

Setting Priorities: What problems need immediate attention? What problems must be addressed on the care plan? What problems must be referred? And in what order do you plan to do all this?

Establishing Goals: Exactly what do you and the patient expect to accomplish, and in what time frame?

Determining Nursing Interventions: What nursing actions and patient activities will help to achieve the goals that you and the patient have set?

Documenting the Nursing Care Plan: Other nurses need to know the plan of care that you have prescribed and the goals you expect to achieve.

☐ **Implementation:** Now is the time to put the plan into action. Putting the plan into action involves the following activities:

Continuing to Collect Information About Your Patient to determine how the patient is responding to your actions and to identify new problems.

Performing the Nursing Interventions and Activities that you prescribed during the planning phase.

Recording (Charting) and Communicating Your Patient's Health Status and Response to Nursing Interventions. You won't be there 24 hours a day, and other nurses and healthcare professionals need to know how the patient is doing and how the plan is working.

☐ **Evaluation:** You and the patient must determine how well the plan has worked and whether you need to make any changes in the plan of care. You must answer the following questions:

Have You and the Patient Achieved the Goals That You Set During the Planning Phase? If so, have any new problems developed that have not been addressed? Could you achieve more than you had originally hoped for? Should you set new goals? What made the plan work? Is there anything you could have done to make it easier?

Have You Only Partially Achieved the Goals, or Perhaps Not at All? If so, why didn't you achieve your goals? Were the goals realistic? Was the patient committed to the goals? Are these goals still important? Did you have enough time? Did other problems arise that impeded your progress? Were your prescribed interventions appropriate? Did you consistently perform the interventions as prescribed? What changes are you going to make?

Display 1-1 summarizes the five steps of the nursing process.

Display 1-1. Steps of the Nursing Process

Assessment—Gathering and examining data.

Diagnosis—Analyzing data to identify strengths and problems.

Planning—Setting goals and developing a plan of action.

Implementation—Putting the plan into action.

Evaluation—Determining if the plan has worked.

To remember the steps of the nursing process, remember the first letter of each of the steps (ADPIE).

How Does the Nursing Process Work?

Using a problem-solving approach is the key to understanding the nursing process. Many of you will recognize the steps listed in Display 1-2 as a common method that you have been using for years to solve the problems that you have encountered in your own lives.

As you can see, the problem-solving method is very evident in the nursing process. Table 1-1 compares the steps of the nursing process and the problem-solving method.

Relationships Among the Steps of the Nursing Process

Assessment and Diagnosis.   As you work with the nursing process, you will find that the first two steps, assessment and diagnosis, overlap significantly. That is, as you gather data, you begin to interpret what the data mean, even though you have not yet "put the whole picture together."

Display 1-2. Steps of the Problem-Solving Method

1. You encounter a problem of some sort and begin to collect information to see if you can understand the problem more clearly.
2. You study the information and identify just what the problem is.
3. You make a plan of action: "This is what I'm going to do about this problem."
4. You carry out the plan of action.
5. You evaluate whether the plan of action is helping to solve the problem. (You ask yourself, "Is this working? Is this problem really better? What else should I be doing to solve this problem?")

Table 1-1. Comparison of Nursing Process and Problem-Solving Method

Nursing Process	Problem-Solving Method
Assessment: Collecting and examining data.	Encountering problem; collecting data
Diagnosis: Analyzing data to identify health problems and strengths.	Analyzing the data to identify exactly what the problem is
Planning: Developing the plan.	Making a plan of action
Implementation: Putting the plan into action.	Putting the plan into action
Evaluation: Determining how well the plan has worked.	Evaluation of results

For example, if a nurse begins an assessment and notes that the patient has an irregular pulse, swollen ankles, and difficulty breathing, she will probably begin to think, "This patient may have a heart problem," as she continues with the assessment.

Some people view diagnosis as a step *within* the assessment phase, or even use the terms interchangeably. They may ask, "What is your *assessment?*" rather than, "What is your *diagnosis?*" For our purposes, we will view assessment and diagnosis as *two separate but closely related and overlapping steps.* Assessment will consist of making sure that you have available all the right pieces of the puzzle that are pertinent to identifying an individual's health status. Diagnosis will consist of the actual "putting together" of the "puzzle pieces" so that a clear picture of the health status becomes evident.

Note how the following diagram shows the close relationship between assessment and diagnosis.

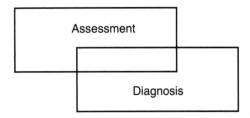

Diagnosis and Planning.   Diagnosis is closely related to planning because the goals that you set during the planning stage are derived *directly from the problems you have diagnosed*. The interventions that are planned are designed to alleviate or prevent the problems, while using identified strengths. For example, if you identify the problem of *Ineffective Individual Coping* and the strength of "has strong family support systems," you might set the following goal: "With the assistance of family support, the individual will demonstrate effective coping." You would then determine a plan that will assist the person to cope more effectively with the help of willing family members. Because of this relationship between *identified problems and strengths* and *establishing goals and determining interventions*, you should be aware that if problem identification is inaccurate, incomplete, or vague, or if you have not taken the time to identify strengths, then it's unlikely that the plan will be effective and efficient.

Diagnosis and planning may overlap because there are times when you have to act quickly, developing and implementing a mental plan of action, before you have time to identify all the problems. For example, if you identified a life-threatening problem, you would need to make a quick mental plan for immediate action. Once the situation was under control, you would then analyze all the data in more depth.

The diagram below shows the relationship between diagnosis and planning.

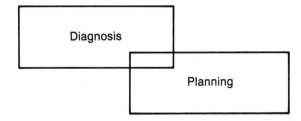

Planning and Implementation.   Planning and implementation are closely related for two reasons:

1. The actions you perform during implementation are guided by the plan that you have developed.

2. As already mentioned above, there may be times when you'll have to plan and implement nursing actions quickly, before the entire plan is developed.

The diagram below shows the relationship between planning and implementation.

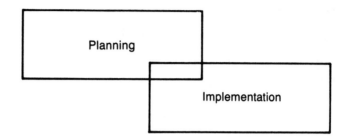

Evaluation and the Other Steps in the Nursing Process.   Evaluation is clearly related to the planning stage because, assuming your diagnoses were accurate and your goals appropriate, the ultimate question to be answered during this phase is, "Have we achieved the goals we set during the planning phase?" However, since we cannot just *assume* that the diagnoses are accurate and the goals are appropriate, and we need to identify things that helped or hindered progress, evaluation involves all of the following:

☐ Performing a complete assessment to determine the client's health status *today* and to make sure that you aren't missing any data

☐ Checking to be sure that your diagnoses are accurate and complete (that you have correctly named the problems and have not missed any)

☐ Making sure that you have set forth an effective plan of care (that the goals and interventions were appropriate, and that you used and reinforced strengths)

☐ Determining whether the plan of care was actually implemented, and identifying factors that helped or hindered progress

☐ Modifying or terminating the plan as indicated depending upon the results of the above activities

The diagram on the next page illustrates how evaluation is related to all the previous steps of the nursing process.

Summary.   The nursing process is a five-step cycle of activities that begins with assessment and culminates with evaluation. Note the example below:

☐ **Assessment:** You note that the person complains that his throat and mouth are dry. His temperature is elevated to 100°F. His record shows that he hasn't had anything to drink all morning. He states that he knows he should

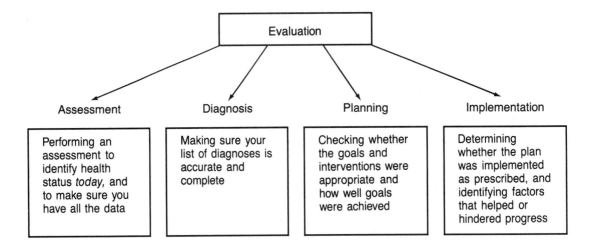

be drinking fluids and wants to drink, but he doesn't like water, especially when warm. He also says he's worried about bothering the nurses.

□ **Diagnosis:** You analyze the above data and identify *Fluid Volume Deficit related to insufficient fluid intake and fever*. You also note that his willingness to increase fluids if they are readily available is a strength.

□ **Planning:** Together with the client, you develop a plan of action by setting a goal of maintaining adequate hydration by his drinking at least 2500 ml/day, and identifying interventions to meet this goal. You document this on the care plan.

□ **Implementation:** You and the other nurses assure that favorite fluids are kept at the bedside on ice. You monitor how the patient is doing in meeting his daily goal. You chart time and amounts of fluid on the intake and output record.

□ **Evaluation:** You perform an assessment and determine whether the patient still has a *Fluid Volume Deficit*. If he is adequately hydrated, and no longer at risk for *Fluid Volume Deficit* (*i.e.*, no longer has a fever), then you terminate the plan and allow him to follow his usual pattern of fluid intake. If he is not adequately hydrated, you must examine the steps above, identify factors that are interfering with goal achievement, and modify the plan as indicated.

Figure 1-1 shows the interrelationship of all the steps.

Why Should We Use the Nursing Process?

Use of the nursing process assists nurses to deliver nursing care in a systematic and organized manner. It guides nurses to take deliberate steps to identify *unique* patient problems, *realistic* goals, and *individualized* interventions. It

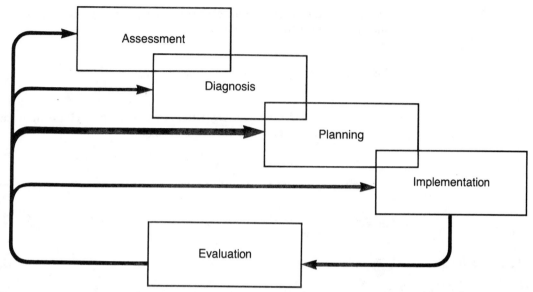

Figure 1-1. *Relationships among the steps of the nursing process. Each step of the nursing process is dependent upon the accuracy of the preceding step. The steps are also overlapping because you may have to move quicker for some problems than others. Evaluation involves examining all the previous steps of the nursing process, but especially focuses upon goal achievement (given that the diagnoses were accurate and goals were appropriate).*

encourages identification and utilization of *client strengths.* Documentation of care plans enhances communication and continuity of care, thus reducing omissions and duplications in patient care.

Unlike the medical model, which focuses on treating the disease, the nursing process is *holistic* in focus, considering both the problems at hand *and* the effect of the problems upon how the person functions as a unique human being. Maintaining this holistic focus complements the work of the physician, ensures that the unique needs are met, and assists nurses to tailor interventions to the individual (and family), rather than the disease.

Display 1-3 gives an example of how a physician and a nurse may focus their assessment, diagnosis, and treatment for the same patient. Display 1-4 summarizes the benefits of using the nursing process.

☐ *Practice Session*　　*Nursing Process Overview*
(Suggested Answers on page 166)
1. List and define the steps of the nursing process.

2. Compare and contrast the nursing treatment plan (*i.e.*, nursing process) and the medical treatment plan.

3. List five advantages of using the nursing process.

4. Discuss the benefits of including patients and significant others in making decisions and developing a nursing care plan.

Display 1-3. Sample Physician's and Nurse's Data for Assessment, Diagnosis, and Treatment

Physician's Data
(*Disease focus*)

"Mrs. Smith has pain and swelling in all joints. Diagnostic studies indicate that she has rheumatoid arthritis. We will start her on course of anti-inflammatories to treat the rheumatoid arthritis."
(*Physician focuses on treating the arthritis.*)

Nurse's Data
(*Holistic focus, considering both problems and their effect upon the patient/family*)

"Mrs. Smith has pain and swelling in all joints, making it difficult to feed and dress herself. She has voiced that it's difficult to feel worthwhile when she can't even feed herself. She states she is depressed because she misses seeing her two small children. We need to develop a plan to help her cope with the pain, to assist her with feeding and dressing, to work through feelings of low self-esteem, and for special visitations with the children."
(*Nurse focuses on the effect of the pain and swelling upon Mrs. Smith as a biopsychosocial individual.*)

Display 1-4. Benefits of Using the Nursing Process

☐ Provides an organized method of giving nursing care
☐ Prevents omissions and unnecessary repetitions
☐ Helps nurses to tailor-make interventions for the individual (not the disease)
☐ Helps patients and families realize that their input is important and that their strong points are assets
☐ Promotes flexibility and independent thinking
☐ Provides for better communication
☐ Helps nurses have the satisfaction of getting results

Key Points　Nursing Process Overview

1. The steps of the nursing process can be remembered by using the mnemonic ADPIE (pronounced ăd'pī): *A*ssessment, *D*iagnosis, *P*lanning, *I*mplementation, *E*valuation.

2. Use of the nursing process guides nurses to be systematic and methodical in identifying *unique* patient problems, *realistic* goals, and *individualized* interventions that utilize client strengths.

3. Each step of the nursing process is dependent on the accuracy of the step preceding it (*e.g.*, correct diagnosis is dependent on correct assessment data).

4. Unlike the medical model, which focuses upon treating the disease, the nursing process is *holistic in focus*, considering both the problems at hand and the effect of the problems upon how the person functions as a unique human being.

Bibliography

American Nurses' Association (1973) *Standards of Nursing Practice*. Kansas City, MO.

American Nurses' Association (1980) *Nursing: A Social Policy Statement*. Kansas City, MO.

Carpenito, L. (1987) *Nursing Diagnosis: Application to Clinical Practice*. 2nd ed. Philadelphia: JB Lippincott.

Gordon, M. (1982) *Nursing Diagnosis: Process and Application*. New York: McGraw-Hill.

Griffith, J. and Christensen, P. (1982) *Nursing Process: Application of Theories, Frameworks and Models*. St Louis: CV Mosby.

Harris, R. (1981) A strong vote for the nursing process. *Am. J. Nurs.* 81:1999–2001.

Soares, C. (1978) Nursing and medical diagnoses: A comparison of variant and essential features. In Chaska, N. (ed): *The Nursing Profession: Views Through the Mist*. New York: McGraw-Hill.

Taylor, C., Lillis, C., and LeMone, P. (1989) *Fundamentals of Nursing: The Art and Science of Nursing Care*. Philadelphia: JB Lippincott.

Ziegler, S., Vaughan-Wroble, B., and Erlen, J. (1986) *Nursing Process, Nursing Diagnosis, Nursing Knowledge: Avenues to Autonomy*. Norwalk, CT: Appleton-Lange.

☑ Collecting Data
☑ Validating Data
☑ Organizing Data
☑ Identifying Patterns
☑ Communicating/Recording Data

2
Assessment

Standard I: *The collection of data about the health status of the client/patient is systematic and continuous. The data are accessible, communicated, and recorded.**

*Abstracted from Standards of Nursing Practice. Copyright American Nurses' Association, 1973

Glossary

Baseline Data Information that describes the status of a problem before treatment began.

Cue(s) Pieces of data that prompt you to suspect a health problem (*i.e.,* *abnormal* objective and subjective data).

Data Base Assessment Comprehensive assessment that is usually completed upon initial contact with the patient to gather information about all aspects of the patient's health.

Focus Assessment Nursing assessment that focuses on gathering more information about a specific problem.

Inference How someone *perceives or interprets* a cue. (*e.g.,* one person may perceive an individual's silence as acceptance, while another may interpret it as defiance, depending on judgment)

Objective Data Information that is concretely *observable* (*i.e.,* information that can be readily and surely seen with the eye [observation], felt with the hand [palpation/percussion], heard with the ear [auscultation], tasted or smelled). Some examples are vital signs; numerical lab reports, such as a blood sugar of 115; diagnostic studies, such as electrocardiograms and x-rays; a limb that is swollen; definite colors such as red or blue.

Subjective Data Information that the patient or client actually tells the nurse during the nursing assessment (usually charted as "Patient states . . . .").

Validation The process of making sure the information or data you have collected is factual or true.

Assessment: Collecting and Examining Data

Assessment is the first step of the nursing process: that first stage of problem identification when you gather information to make sure that "all the necessary pieces of the puzzle" are available to put together a clear picture of the client's health status. Unlike the second step, diagnosis, when you actually "put together the puzzle" and identify health problems, the assessment phase deals mostly with *collecting the "puzzle pieces"* (*i.e., data*), *examining what they look like, and determining where they might fit into the picture.* Because *all* nursing decisions and interventions are based on the information gathered during this phase, you should consider this step to be very important. During the assessment phase you should be gathering as much pertinent information about the patient as possible. This process of gathering information will include the following activities:

☐ **Collecting Data:** Gathering information about the patient or client

☐ **Validating Data:** Making sure that you know which data are actually fact and which data are questionable

☐ **Organizing Data:** Clustering the data into groups of information that will help you to identify patterns of health or disease

☐ **Identifying Patterns:** Making an initial impression about patterns of information, and gathering additional data to fill in the gaps to describe more clearly what the data mean

☐ **Communicating/Recording Data:** Reporting significant data to expedite treatment, and completing the data base

Collecting Data

Data collection begins with the client's first encounter with the healthcare system. (This could happen on an outpatient basis, but for our purposes we will assume it is a hospital admission.) At the time of admission, a comprehensive nursing assessment is accomplished, and pertinent data are documented on the chart and on the nursing care plan. Data collection *continues throughout the patient's hospital stay* as changes occur and new information is presented.

Let's take a look at this process of data collection and consider the resources and methods that you should be using to gather information about the health state of a given individual.

What Resources Should Be Used to Gather Data?

When you gather data, you should use as many appropriate resources as possible. However, it is important to remember that *the patient should be considered the primary source of information*. You will be gathering information from medical records, nursing records, the patient's family, other professionals who are working with the patient, and literature that you have found concerning the patient's problems. All of these resources will be valuable, but your direct examination and interview of the patient is likely to offer some of the most significant pieces of information.

The following summarizes the resources for gathering data.

☐ Patient/client (primary source)

☐ Family/significant others

☐ Nursing records

☐ Medical records

☐ Verbal/written consultations (with other healthcare professionals)

☐ Records of diagnostic studies

☐ Relevant literature

How Should Data Be Gathered?

Comprehensive data collection usually occurs in three phases. First, you gather information before you actually see the patient. (In order to keep an open mind, many diagnosticians ask only to know the patient's name, age, and sex before going in to meet the patient. Others find it helpful to read patient records before meeting the patient, depending upon the situation.) Secondly, you perform a nursing assessment by interviewing, examining, and observing the patient. Finally, you review the resources that you have used, and note if there are other resources that may offer additional information. If you have missed a pertinent resource, you should take the time to locate it and gather more data to be sure that you've been thorough.

Types of Nursing Assessment

Comprehensive data collection includes two types of nursing assessment:

☐ **Data Base Nursing Assessment:** Performed upon *initial contact* with the patient to gather information about *all* aspects of the patient's health status. This information (called *baseline data*) tells you how the patient is *today*, before interventions begin, and will be the basis for identifying strengths and problems.

☐ **Focus Assessment:** Performed to focus on the status of an actual or potential problem.

Data Base Nursing Assessment.   Data base assessment should be planned, systematic, and comprehensive to ensure that all pertinent information is obtained. You will find that your method of data collection will be influenced by how you are educated and by the assessment tool that you're using. In recent years, most schools and facilities have changed the focus of their data base assessment tools from a medical model (disease-oriented) to a nursing model (holistic, human response-oriented). Using a data base form that is designed to gather information according to a *nursing model* is very important. This is because a data base that is organized primarily on the medical model will help you to gather information only about *medical* problems. Without a *holistic nursing focus,* you are likely to miss important information about how the person functions as a biopsychosocial human being. It is this type of data, *how the person lives his or her daily life,* that will be crucial to consider later, when you identify nursing diagnoses.

There are several ways of organizing a nursing data base to maintain a *nursing focus.* Examples of comprehensive nursing data base tools can be found on pages 17–27. Figures 2-1 through 2-3 provide examples of data base tools that are organized according to Gordon's Functional Health Patterns (Fig. 2-1), Orem's Theory of Self Care (Fig. 2-2), and to meet the specific needs of a given hospital (Fig. 2-3). Other popular models that are used to guide a

(Text continues on page 28)

Figure 2-1. *Data base assessment form organized according to Gordon's functional health patterns. (Reprinted with permission from the Bronson Methodist Hospital, Kalamazoo, Michigan)*

BRONSON METHODIST HOSPITAL
Kalamazoo, Michigan

Medical/Surgical–Critical Care Admission Assessment

A. **DEMOGRAPHIC DATA**

Name: _____

Prefers to be called: _____ Age: _____

Date: _____ Time of arrival to unit: _____

Mode of admission: _____

I.D. bracelet on and coincides with addressograph: ☐ Yes ☐ No Information given by: _____

If unable to reach next of kin/legal guardian, contact: _____ Phone: _____

Valuables (list and state disposition): _____

Admitted from: ☐ Home ☐ Nursing Home ☐ Assisted Living ☐ Foster Care ☐ Senior Citizens' Apartments ☐ Other

Facility Name: _____ Adm. Medical Diagnosis: _____

B. **VITAL SIGNS**

Ht: _____ Wt: _____ Kg

Temp: _____ ☐ Oral ☐ Ax. ☐ Rectal

Pulse: _____ ☐ Reg. ☐ Irreg.

Resp.: _____ ☐ Reg. ☐ Irreg.

BP: Left: _____

☐ Lying ☐ Sitting ☐ Standing

Right: _____

☐ Lying ☐ Sitting ☐ Standing

C. **ORIENTATION TO UNIT**

(The following have been explained):

Call system/bed–bathroom	☐ Yes ☐ N/A	Floor restrictions	☐ Yes ☐ N/A
Bed operation/siderails	☐ Yes ☐ N/A	Visitation Policy	☐ Yes ☐ N/A
Bathroom/bedpan–urinal	☐ Yes ☐ N/A	Lounge	☐ Yes ☐ N/A
TV/CH2/telephone	☐ Yes ☐ N/A	Newspaper/mail	☐ Yes ☐ N/A
Meal/cafeteria hours	☐ Yes ☐ N/A	Siderails policy	☐ Yes ☐ N/A
Smoking policy	☐ Yes ☐ N/A	Chaplain services	☐ Yes ☐ N/A

Signature: _____

D. **Health Patterns Assessment:** Complete information, **including patient's words.** Indicate N/A if non-applicable. Circle, code, or check all other findings as appropriate.

1. **HEALTH PERCEPTION/HEALTH MANAGEMENT**

Reason for hospitalization/chief complaint: _____

Recent illness/exposure to communicable disease: _____

Previous hospitalizations/surgeries: _____

What other health problems have you had? _____

Things done to manage health: _____

Statement of patient's general appearance (include condition of hair, skin, nails): _____

Tobacco use: ☐ Yes ☐ No ☐ Used to smoke: _____

EtOH use: _____

Allergies: ☐ Yes (list with reaction experienced) ☐ No

Food: _____

Medications/anesthetics: _____

Other (e.g., wool, tape, pollens): _____

FORM 102 (Revised 10/84) — Page 1

(Continued)

Figure 2-1. *(Continued)*

Patient's Name: _____ Hospital No.: _____ Date: _____

Medications: (e.g., prescript., non-prescript.) ☐ Yes ☐ No Did you bring? ☐ Yes ☐ No Taken home? ☐ Yes ☐ No ☐ N/A

NAME	DOSE	SCHEDULE	REASON	PRESCRIBING PHYSICIAN

Have you been taking your medication(s) as prescribed? _____

OTHER PERTINENT DATA: _____ | initials

2. Special diet? _____ Supplements: _____

NUTRITION / METABOLIC

Pattern of daily food/fluid intake: _____

Appetite: _____ Wt. loss/gain: _____

Nausea/Vomiting: _____

GI pain: _____

Condition of oral mucous membranes: _____

Dental condition: _____ Dentures: ☐ Upper ☐ Lower ☐ Partial ☐ N/A

Skin: ☐ Warm ☐ Dry ☐ Cool ☐ Moist ☐ Other: _____

Turgor: ☐ Supple ☐ Firm ☐ Fragile ☐ Dehydrated ☐ Other: _____

Color: ☐ Pink ☐ Pale ☐ Dusky ☐ Cyanotic ☐ Jaundiced ☐ Mottled ☐ Other: ____

Edema: _____

Wounds/drains/dressings: _____

Skin problems (description and location): _____

_____ ☐ N/A

I.V.'s: _____

OTHER PERTINENT DATA: _____ | initials

3. Abd. tenderness/guarding/distention: _____ Stoma (type): _____

ELIMINATION

Bowel sounds: _____

Any problems with hemorrhoids/involuntary stool? _____

Usual bowel pattern (frequency, character, consistency, etc.): _____ Date of last BM: _____

If problem, describe: _____

Use of anything to manage bowels (e.g., laxatives, enemas, suppositories, "home remedies", anti-diarrheals): ____

Usual urinary pattern (frequency, character, amount, incontinence, nocturia, etc.): ____

_____ Last void (time): _____

If problem, describe: _____

Perspiration/nocturnal sweats: _____

OTHER PERTINENT DATA: _____ | initials

FOHM 102 (Revised 10/84) — Page 2

(Continued)

4.

CARDIO-VASCULAR STATUS

Peripheral pulses: _____
_____ ☐ N/A
Neurovascular check (e.g., capillary refill): _____
_____
Chest pain/radiation: _____
_____
Jugular vein distention: ☐ Yes ☐ No
Hx of murmur: ☐ Yes ☐ No
Pacemaker: ☐ Yes ☐ No
Presence of A-V Shunt: _____ ☐ No
Arterio-venous bruit: _____ ☐ N/A
Monitor/rhythm: _____ ☐ N/A
Hemodynamic monitoring: _____ ☐ N/A

RESPIRATORY STATUS

Respiratory pattern: ☐ No problem ☐ Dyspnea ☐ Nocturnal Dyspnea ☐ S.O.B. at rest
☐ S.O.B. on exertion: _____ ☐ Other: _____
Lung sounds: _____ Use of accessory muscles? ☐ Yes ☐ No
Cough/production: _____ O_2 supplement: _____ ☐ N/A
Resp. tubes (e.g., ET, trach, chest/describe secretions/drainage): _____
_____ ☐ N/A
Ventilatory assistance: _____ ☐ N/A

ACTIVITIES OF DAILY LIVING/MOBILITY STATUS

Use the **Activity Level Code** below to assess admission statuses:

	ADL Status		**Mobility Status**
0-total independence	Feeding _____	Meal Preparation _____	Bed mobility _____
1-assist with device	Bathing _____	Cleaning _____	Cart transfer _____
2-assist with person	Dressing _____	Shopping _____	Chair/toilet transfer _____
3-assist with device & person	Grooming _____	Laundry _____	Ambulation _____
4-total dependence	Toileting _____	Other _____	R.O.M. _____

Handedness: ☐ Right ☐ Left
Able to use? ☐ Yes ☐ No
Reasons for ADL/Mobility limitations: _____
_____ ☐ N/A
Devices used for assist: _____ ☐ N/A
Do you need assistance with transportation? ☐ Yes ☐ No If "Yes", specify: _____
Where do you plan to be discharged? _____ Will you need assistance? ☐ Yes ☐ No
If "Yes", describe: _____
OTHER PERTINENT DATA: _____
_____
| initials |

5.

REFLEXES

Level of consciousness: _____ Oriented to: ☐ Person ☐ Place ☐ Time
Behaviors (describe): _____
Hx of epilepsy/seizures/Parkinson's, etc.: _____

Reflexes: ☐ No problem ☐ Problem (If "No problem", do not complete this section.)
Eyes: Pupil size: r_____ l_____ Equal? ☐ Yes ☐ No Reaction to light: r_____ l_____
Accommodation: r_____ l_____ Deviation: _____
Handgrasp: r_____ l_____ Gag: _____ Swallow: _____
Movement of extremities: _____

SENSORIUM

Eyes/sight: ☐ No problem ☐ Deficit: _____ Aid: _____
Ears/hearing: ☐ No problem ☐ Deficit: _____ Aid: _____
Nose/smell: ☐ No problem ☐ Deficit: _____
Tongue/taste: ☐ No problem ☐ Deficit: _____
Skin/touch: ☐ No problem ☐ Deficit: _____
Numbness/tingling: ☐ No problem ☐ Deficit: _____
Dizziness: ☐ No problem ☐ Deficit: _____

(vertical labels: ACTIVITY / EXERCISE, COGNITIVE / PERCEPTUAL)

FORM 102 (Revised 10/84) — Page 3

(Continued)

Figure 2-1. (Continued)

Patient's Name: _____ Hospital No.: _____ Date: _____

COGNITIVE/PERCEPTUAL

PAIN

Pain: □ No problem □ Problem (If "No problem", do not complete this section.)
If "Problem", describe location, type, intensity, onset, duration: _____
_____
_____
Methods of pain management: _____

COGNITION

Primary language: _____ Speech deficit: _____ Aid: _____
Any learning difficulties? _____
OTHER PERTINENT DATA: _____
_____ | initials |

6.

SLEEP/REST

Usual sleep/rest pattern: _____
Adequate? □ Yes □ No Factors affecting sleep/rest: _____
Methods to promote sleep: _____
Hx of sleep disturbances: _____
OTHER PERTINENT DATA: _____ | initials |

7.

SELF–PERCEPTION SELF–CONCEPT

Are there any ways you feel differently about yourself since you've been ill/hospitalized? _____
_____
_____
Description of non-verbal behaviors: _____
OTHER PERTINENT DATA: _____ | initials |

8.

ROLE/RELATIONSHIP

Marital status: _____ Children: _____
Do you live? □ Alone □ With family □ Other: _____
Family feelings regarding hospitalization: _____
Who are the people that will help you most at this time? _____
Are you presently employed? □ Yes □ No Occupation: _____ □ N/A
Are you presently in school? □ Yes □ No Will illness/hospitalization interfere? _____ □ N/A
Upon discharge, if necessary, will you be able to afford?
          Medications: □ Yes □ No   Supplies: □ Yes □ No   Medical Care: □ Yes □ No
OTHER PERTINENT DATA _____
_____ | initials |

9.

SEXUALITY/REPRODUCTIVE

Female: □ N/A   Menopausal: □ Yes □ No   Menstrual pattern: _____ □ N/A
  Problems/changes: _____
  Date of L.N.M.P. _____ □ N/A Possibly pregnant? □ Yes □ No □ N/A
  Pregnancy history: _____
  Use of birth control measure □ Yes □ No □ N/A Type: _____
    Any problems with use? _____
  Monthly self-breast exam? □ Yes □ No □ N/A
  Vaginal discharge/bleeding/lesions: _____
    Receiving medical attention? □ Yes □ No □ N/A
  OTHER PERTINENT DATA: _____ | initials |

Male: □ N/A   Prostate problems? _____
Monthly self-testicular exam? □ Yes □ No □ N/A
Penile discharge/bleeding/lesions: _____
  Receiving medical attention? □ Yes □ No □ N/A
  OTHER PERTINENT DATA: _____ | initials |

FORM 102 (Revised 10/84) — Page 4

(Continued)

10. Have you experienced any recent stressful situations in addition to your
illness/hospitalization? ☐ Yes ☐ No
If "Yes", please describe briefly: _____
_____
_____
_____

Are there any ways we can be of assistance? _____
_____

How do you usually manage stresses? _____
_____
_____

What do you do for relaxation? _____

Support groups/counselling resources used: _____
Were they helpful? _____ ☐ N/A
OTHER PERTINENT DATA: _____
_____

| | initials |

COPING/STRESS

11. Will illness/hospitalization interfere with any of the following?
Spiritual or religious practices? ☐ Yes ☐ No
Cultural beliefs or practices? ☐ Yes ☐ No
Familial traditions? ☐ Yes ☐ No
If "Yes", to any of the above, please describe briefly: _____
_____
_____
_____
_____

Would you like your clergy or hospital chaplain to be contacted? ☐ Yes ☐ No ☐ N/A
OTHER PERTINENT DATA: _____
_____

| | initials |

VALUE/BELIEF

E. Include: a. Possible nursing diagnostic concept labels to consider for care planning.
        b. Possible referral resources to consider for discharge planning needs.
        c. Other pertinent information

_____
_____
_____
_____
_____
_____
_____
_____
_____
_____
_____
_____
_____

| | initials |

IMPRESSIONS

DATE	TIME	INITIALS	SIGNATURES	
_____	_____	_____	_____	(1st Adm. R.N.)
_____	_____	_____	_____	(2nd Adm. R.N.)
_____	_____	_____	_____	(3rd Adm. R.N.)
_____	_____	_____	_____	(4th Adm. R.N.)

FORM 102 (Revised 10/84) — Page 5 .

Figure 2-2. *Data base assessment form organized according to Orem's theory of self-care. (Reprinted with permission from Holy Family College Department of Nursing, Philadelphia, Pennsylvania)*

Nursing History

I. Client profile
  A. Personal characteristics
    1. Name
    2. Age
    3. Sex
    4. Marital status
    5. Ethnic orientation
    6. Relgious orientation
    7. Educational level
    8. Language
    9. Occupational history (type of job, duration)
    10. Interest, hobbies, recreational activities
  B. Current health orientation
    1. What do you consider to be healthy about you?
    2. What are your health goals?
  C. Family characteristics
    1. Family members/significant others (age, relationship to client)
    2. Type of family form
    3. Family structure
      a. Role structure
      b. Value systems
      c. Communication pattern
      d. Power structure
    4. Family function
      a. Affective function
      b. Socialization and social placement function
      c. Reproductive function
      d. Family coping function
      e. Economic function
      f. Provision of physical necessities
  D. Environmental characteristics
    1. Physical setting: home (characteristics, safety hazards, spatial adequacy, provision of privacy)
    2. Physical setting: neighborhood and community, including geographic mobility patterns; presence of environmental hazards
    3. Associations and transactions of the family with the community, and perception and feelings about neighborhood and community; include accessibility of health-care facilities, human services
II. Universal self-care requisites
  A. Air
    1. Health habits
      a. Hygiene (bathing and grooming practices, oral hygiene, feminine hygiene, special cultural practices)
      b. Patterns of oxygenation (special aids)
    2. Review of systems
      a. Skin: rashes, pruritis, scaling, lesions, turgor, skin growths, tumors, masses, pigmentation changes or discoloration
      b. Hair: changes in amount, texture, character; alopecia, use of dyes
      c. Nails: changes in appearance, texture, capillary refill
      d. Breast: pain, skin changes, lesions, dimpling, lumps, nipple discharge, mastectomy

(Continued)

Figure 2-2.   *(Continued)*

    e. Respiratory system: nose (pain or trauma, olfaction, sensitivity, epistaxis, discharge); shortness of breath, dyspnea, chronic cough, sputum production, hemoptysis; history of asthma, wheezing, or noise with breathin

    f. Cardiovascular system: palpitations, heart murmur, varicose veins, history of heart disease; hypertension, chest pain, orthopnea

    g. Peripheral vascular system: coldness, numbness, discoloration, peripheral edema, intermittent claudication

B. Water
  1. Health habits
    a. Patterns of fluid intake
    b. Fluid likes/dislikes
    c. Fluid temperature preferences
  2. Review of systems
    a. Hydration: dehydration, excessive dryness, sweating; odors, edema, polydipsia
    b. Parenteral fluids (IV blood administration, hyperalimentation)

C. Food
  1. Health habits
    a. 24-hour diet recall
    b. Foods likes and dislikes
    c. Dietary modifications (cultural, religious, medical)
    d. Food preparation
    e. Meal environment
    f. Food budgeting
    g. Food supplements (vitamins, minerals, fluorinated water supply)
    h. Weight gain/loss patterns
    i. Problems related to ingestion/digestion (special aids)
    j. Related prescribed or patent medicines
  2. Review of systems
    a. Mouth: teeth, gums, tongue, buccae, chewing difficulty
    b. Throat: pain, lesions, dysarthria, dysphagia, history of strep infections
    c. Gastrointestinal system: pain, anorexia, nausea/vomiting, acid indigestion, ulcer history, polyphagia, present height–weight status

D. Elimination
  1. Health habits
    a. Daily patterns (bladder, bowel)
    b. Aids (fluids, foods, medications, enemas)
  2. Review of systems
    a. Bladder: polyuria, oliguria, dysuria, nocturia, incontinence, difficulty stopping or starting stream, force of stream, dribbling, pain or burning on urination, urinary tract infections
    b. Bowel: pain, diarrhea, constipation (acute or chronic), flatulence, hemorrhoids, stool characteristics (color, consistency, amount)
    c. Surgical opening: draining wounds, ostomies
    d. Genitalia: perineal rashes and irritations, lesions, unusual discharge (amount, color, consistency)

E. Activity and rest
  1. Health habits
    a. Activity patterns: means of ambulation (safety concerns, aids); level of activity (home, work, leisure); regular exercise program
    b. Sleep/rest patterns: circadian rhythms; time and duration of sleep; use of supportive aids (sedatives, alcohol, pillows), devices (reading, music)

(Continued)

Figure 2-2. *(Continued)*

2. Review of systems
   a. Musculoskeletal system: muscle strength/weakness, muscle tone, range of motion, pain, fatigue, swelling, stiffness, contractures
   b. Neurological system: numbness, tingling; discrimination between heat, cold, and touch; unusual movements (tremors, seizures); paralysis; dizziness, headache, loss of consciousness, memory changes; intolerance to heat and cold
F. Solitude and social interaction
  1. Health habits
   a. Communication
   b. Social interactions
   c. Sexuality: attitudes toward own sexuality (femininity/masculinity), sexual orientation, frequency of sexual activity, satisfaction with sexual activity, contraceptive measures
   d. Solitude: opportunities and selected activities during solitude
  2. Review of systems
   a. Ear: pain, discharge, tinnitus, decrease/increase inhearing, use of hearing aids
   b. Eye: pain, discharge, vision, corrective lenses, blurred vision, diplopia, night blindness, color vision
   c. Reproductive system:
    Male: number of offspring, infertility, venereal disease.
    Female: age of menarche, number of days in cycle, type and amount of flow, premenstrual tension, dysmenorrhea/menorrhagia, polymenorrhagia, intermenstrual metrorrhagia, history of pregnancies, number of live births, number of abortions (less than 20 weeks gestation), number of still births, number of neonatal deaths, high-risk pregnancies, infertility, age of menopause
G. Hazards to human life, human functioning, and human well-being
  1. Personal safety practices
  2. Social habits (drugs, alcohol, tobacco, coffee–tea–coke; specify level of use)
H. Normalcy: promotion of human functioning and development within social groups in accord with human potential, known limitations, and the human desire to be normal
  1. Health habits
   a. health resources used (medical, dental, vision and hearing, screening programs, immunizations, counseling)
   b. Personal health practices (stress/anxiety management, meditation, relaxation techniques; self-breast exam, testicular exam)
  2. Self concept/image
   a. Body image (appearance, boundaries, limits, inner structure)
   b. Mental health:
    (1) attitude
    (2) affect/mood
    (3) thought processes (logical, coherent, perceptual)
    (4) sensorium and reasoning (levels of consciousness, orientation, memory, calculation, abstract thinking, judgment/insight, intelligence
    (5) locus of control
    (6) potential for danger (harm to self/others)
   c. Spirituality
III. Developmental self-care requisites
  A. Life-cycle stage and related concerns (neonatal, infancy, toddler, pre-school, school age, adolescence, early adulthood, middle adulthood, childbearing, late adulthood)
  B. Psychosexual stage (Freud)
  C. Psychosocial stage (Erikson)
  D. Intellectual stage (Piaget)
  E. Moral stage (Kohlburg)
  F. Conditions that promote or prevent normal development (life events, poor health, education)

(Continued)

Figure 2-2.   *(Continued)*

IV. Health deviation self-care requisites
   A. Present deviation
      1. Perception of deviation
         a. Reason for contact
         b. Understanding of this current alteration in health status
         c. Feelings about present health status
         d. Specific concerns
      2. Coping mechanisms
         a. Past use of coping mechanisms to deal with similar alterations
         b. Current repertoire of coping mechanisms and their adequacy
         c. Concurrent stresses (life events)
      3. Effects of deviation on life styles
         a. Psychological   c. Financial
         b. Physiological
   B. Past history of health deviations
      1. Adult illness
      2. Childhood illness
      3. Accidents/injuries
      4. Hospitalizations
      5. Allergies
         a. Drugs   c. Other
         b. Food
      6. Medications
         a. Prescription   b. Self-prescribed
   C. Family health history
      1. Relatives living or dead with similar health deviations
      2. Presence of any hereditary diseases (diabetes, hypertension, heart disease)

Figure 2-3. *Sample data base assessment form (WNL = within normal limits).*
(Courtesy of the Wilmington Medical Center, Wilmington, Delaware)

Adult Nursing History
Admission Data Base

Date_____   Arrival Time_____

Arrived via: Ambulatory   Wheelchair   Stretcher
Admitted: From_____To_____
Information obtained from: Patient   Family (specify)_____ Other (specify)_____
Occupation_____ Members of household (specify)_____

Deferred | **I. Communications Status**
Level of consciousness: Alert   Drowsy   Confused   Nonresponsive
Oriented   Yes   No   Specify_____
Cooperative   Yes   No   Specify_____
Language spoken: English   Spanish   Other (specify)_____
Speech: Clear   Slurred   Aphasic   Garbled   Unable to speak
Ability to express self verbally: Yes   No
Ability to communicate: Appropriate   Inappropriate
Hearing: WNL   Impaired   Deaf   Corrected   Lip-reads
Vision: WNL   Impaired   Blind   Corrected
Vertigo: Yes   No   Specify_____

II. History
Reason for admission (patient's statement) _____
_____.
What does patient expect from this hospitalization? _____
_____.

Previous hospital experience?   Yes   No
Existing medical problems:
  Diabetes   Cardiac disease   Arthritis   CVA   Other _____
  Hypertension   Cancer   Respiratory   Renal   _____
Allergies: None known
  Medications   Yes   No   Specify_____Reaction_____
  Food   Yes   No   Specify_____Reaction_____
  Other _____
Prostheses, appliances, or other devices:
  False eye   Braces   Dentures   Eyeglasses
  Artificial limbs   Hearing aid   Contact lenses   Cane
  Pacemaker   Wig   Walker   Ostomy
  Other (specify) _____
Medications (prescription, over-the-counter)?   Yes   No   If yes, list below
  Medicine   Dose   Reason   With patient   Last dose   Prescribing physician
  _____
  _____
  _____
  _____
  _____
  _____

(Continued)

Figure 2-3. (Continued)

Deferred | III. **Functional Status** □ Bedrest □ BRP □ Up ad lib □ Immobile
□ Right-handed □ Left-handed □ Ambidextrous

Motor Function: Specify
R Arm__WNL__Amputated__Spastic__Flaccid__Paresis__Paralysis__Other_____
L Arm__WNL__Amputated__Spastic__Flaccid__Paresis__Paralysis__Other_____
R Leg__WNL__Amputated__Spastic__Flaccid__Paresis__Paralysis__Other_____
L Leg__WNL__Amputated__Spastic__Flaccid__Paresis__Paralysis__Other_____

Patient's ability to ambulate: □ Independent □ Assistance needed _____
        Gait: □ Stable □ Unstable
Bathe: □ Independent □ Assistance needed_____
Dress: □ Independent □ Assistance needed_____
Toilet: □ Independent □ Assistance needed_____
Eat: □ Independent □ Assistance needed_____
  Swallow liquids □ Yes □ No   Swallow solids □ Yes □ No
  Chew □ Yes □ No

Does the patient have problems/difficulty in:
Sleeping □ Yes □ No Specify_____
Eating □ Yes □ No Specify_____
Urination □ Yes □ No Specify_____
Defecation □ Yes □ No Specify_____

IV. **Physical Assessment**
Vital signs: Temp_____BP_____Weight_____Height_____
Pulse_____Strong_____Weak_____Regular_____Irregular_____
Pedal pulse_____Deferred_____
Pupils: □ Equal □ Unequal

Left: •••●●● Reactive to light
           Left □ Yes □ No Specify_____
Right: •••●●● Right □ Yes □ No Specify_____

Eyes: □ Clear □ Draining □ Reddened □ Other
Mouth: Gums □ WNL □ White plaques □ Lesions □ Other _____
      Teeth □ WNL □ Loose □ Other_____

Skin:
Color □ WNL □ Pale □ Cyanotic □ Ashen □ Jaundice □ Other _____
Temperature □ Warm □ Cool Turgor: □ WNL □ Poor
Edema □ No □ Yes Description/location _____
Lesions □ None □ Yes Description/location _____
Decubitus □ None □ Yes Description/location _____
Bruises □ None □ Yes Description/location _____
Reddened □ No □ Yes Description/location _____
Pruritus □ No □ Yes Description/location _____

Respiratory rate _____
Quality: □ WNL □ Shallow □ Rapid □ Labored □ Other _____
Auscultation: Specify
Upper right lobes □ WNL □ Decreased □ Absent □ Abnormal sounds _____
Upper left lobes □ WNL □ Decreased □ Absent □ Abnormal sounds _____
Lower right lobes □ WNL □ Decreased □ Absent □ Abnormal sounds _____
Lower left lobes □ WNL □ Decreased □ Absent □ Abnormal sounds _____
Is patient aware of diagnosis? □ Yes □ No □ Dx not established
What is the person most concerned about? _____
Summary Statement: _____
_____
_____
_____
_____

Date_____Time_____ □ am
                     □ pm _____RN

nursing assessment include Roy's Adaptation Model, Roger's Unitary Man Model, King's Systems Model, Yura and Walsh's Needs Model, and Chrisman and Fowler's Systems-in-Change Model (see Bibliography at end of chapter). You will note that although these tools vary, they all are well organized, comprehensive and *holistic* in focus. Following this type of tool consistently will help you become organized, systematic, and comprehensive.

Focus Assessment.   Focus assessment is used to gather information that is specific to determining the status of an actual or potential problem. You perform a focus assessment to *focus in* on actual and potential problems. For example, suppose during a data base assessment, the patient expresses that he has "trouble with balance from time to time." You would have to focus on assessing the problem of balance by asking more questions about what he means by "having trouble with balance from time to time" (and if appropriate, by observing his gait).

Focus assessment is the main method for ongoing assessment. That is, you have identified an actual or potential problem, and now you will have to perform periodic focus assessments to monitor its status. When you perform a focus assessment, you should ask yourself the following questions:

☐ Are there observable signs and symptoms that demonstrate that the problem exists *right now?* (If so, what are they? Are they getting better, worse, or staying the same?)

☐ Are there factors contributing to the problem that can be reduced, controlled, or eliminated to alleviate or prevent the problem?

☐ How does the person feel about managing or preventing the problem? Is he able to verbalize how to manage or prevent the problem?

Display 2-1 shows how these questions may be applied to the problem of constipation.

Display 2-1. Focus Assessment For Constipation

1. Are there observable signs and symptoms of constipation? (*i.e.,* hard, dry stool; abdominal cramping; no recent bowel movement; difficulty passing the stool)? Are these symptoms getting better, worse, or staying the same?

2. Are there factors contributing to constipation (poor diet, lack of fluid intake, medications, immobility) that can be modified to alleviate or prevent the constipation?

3. How does the person feel about managing or preventing constipation? Is he able to relate how to manage or prevent constipation?

The Nursing Interview and Physical Assessment

Even though nursing data base forms are helpful tools in guiding a nursing assessment, the success of your efforts to identify patterns of health or illness will depend upon your skill in performing an interview and physical examination. And you must become skilled at doing *both* because each of these activities complements and clarifies the other. For example, consider the following situations that show how information gained from physical examination complements and clarifies information gathered from the nursing interview.

Situation 1

You interview someone who tells you, "I feel like my breathing isn't quite right, but I can't explain exactly what I mean." You then take a stethoscope and listen to his lungs. What you hear (whether the lung sounds are normal or abnormal) gives you additional information that complements and clarifies what the patient told you, and helps you determine what is meant by "my breathing isn't quite right." You begin to get a better picture of the problem, because you have two types of data to consider: *what the patient has told you* about his breathing and what *you have observed* about his breathing.

Now consider the next situation, which shows how interviewing techniques can complement and clarify information gained from physical examination.

Situation 2

You perform a physical examination and notice that the individual has a cyst the size of a quarter in the right shoulder area. Although the person did not mention any problems with cysts in an initial interview, you specifically ask whether this is something new. The reply may help you determine if this is an acute problem that needs to be studied, or whether the patient simply forgot to mention that this is a problem that has already been evaluated.

You can see how vital it is to perform *both* a physical examination and an interview to be sure that you gather all pertinent information. The nursing interview and the nursing physical assessment are two activities that are forever intertwined, and essential to completing a nursing assessment.

The Nursing Interview.   What you see and what you hear during the nursing interview will yield important information for your nursing assessment. The amount of pertinent data collected will depend on your interviewing skills (*i.e.*, your ability to establish rapport, and to observe, listen, and question).

Establishing rapport and learning to observe, listen, and question comes with practice, but the following guidelines for promoting a successful interview will help you to develop these skills.

☐ *Guidelines*　　　　*Promoting a Successful Interview*

How to Establish Rapport

- ☐ **Ensure Privacy.** Provide a quiet, private setting without interruptions or distractions.
- ☐ **Use the Person's Name.** Introduce yourself and show a genuine interest in the individual's well being.
- ☐ **Explain Your Purpose.** Explain that the purpose of asking so many questions is to provide better nursing care by knowing more about the person and his family.
- ☐ **Use Good Eye Contact.** Give the person your full attention.
- ☐ **Don't Hurry.** Rushing may cause the person to feel that you are not interested in hearing what he has to say.

How to Observe

- ☐ **Use Your Senses.** Do you see, hear, or smell anything abnormal?
- ☐ **Notice General Appearance.** Does the person appear well groomed, healthy, well nourished?
- ☐ **Notice Body Language.** Does the person appear comfortable? Nervous? Withdrawn? Apprehensive? What do you see?
- ☐ **Notice Interaction Patterns.** Be aware of the person's responses to your interviewing style (for example, sometimes cultural differences will create communication barriers).

How to Ask Questions

- ☐ **Ask About the Person's Main Problem First.** Asking questions about the problem that made him seek healthcare helps him feel purpose and expedience in your questioning.
- ☐ **Use Terminology that the Person Understands.** Ask the person to repeat what has been said if you think he does not understand.
- ☐ **Use Open-Ended Questions.** Ask questions that require more than a one-word answer. (See Display 2-2 for examples.)
- ☐ **Use Reflection** (restating the person's own words in a question) to encourage him to expand on what has been said. (See Display 2-3 for examples.)
- ☐ **Don't Start with Personal or Delicate Questions.** Hold these questions until you get to know the person.
- ☐ **Defer Questions that Are not Pertinent** if the person is too uncomfortable or upset. Only ask questions that are absolutely necessary.
- ☐ **Use an Organized Assessment Tool to Prevent Omissions.** This is usually provided by the institution, or you can use any of the data base assessment tools shown in this book.

How to Listen

☐ **Be an Active Listener.** A nod or a glance of interest will help to encourage the patient to go on.

☐ **Allow the Person to Finish Sentences.** Be calm and sympathetic, and don't rush him.

☐ **Be Patient if the Person Has a Memory Block.** Give him time, and he may jog his memory when you ask related questions.

☐ **Give Your Full Attention.** Discourage unnecessary interruptions.

☐ **For Clarification, Summarize and Restate What Has Been Said.** This reduces misunderstanding on the part of both the patient and the nurse.

Display 2-2.   Examples of Open-Ended Questions and Closed-Ended Questions

Closed-Ended: "Are you happy about this?"
Open-Ended: "How does this make you feel?"

Closed-Ended: "Do you get along with your husband?"
Open-Ended: "How is your relationship with your husband?"

Closed-Ended: "Does this make you sick to your stomach?"
Open-Ended: "Describe the feeling that you are experiencing."

Display 2-3.   Examples of Reflective Statements

Client states: "Sometimes I'm happy about how things are going, and sometimes I feel that everything is all wrong."
Reflective response: "So you feel happy some of the time, but sometimes things don't seem right?"

Client states: "I wish I could be somewhere else."
Reflective response: " . . . Somewhere else?"

☐ *Practice Session*   *The Nursing Interview*
(Suggested Answers on page 166)

1. **Practice Making Open-Ended Questions.** Rewrite each question below so that it is an open-ended question.

   a. "Are you feeling better?"

    b. "Did you like dinner?"

    c. "Are you happy here?"

    d. "Are you having pain?"

    e. "Are you and your wife happy?"

2. **Practice Clarifying Ideas by Using Reflection and Making Open-Ended Questions.** For each statement below, write a reflective statement and an open-Ended question that would help you to clarify what has been said.
   a. "I've been sick off and on for a month."

   b. "Nothing ever goes right for me."

   c. "I seem to have a pain in my side that comes and goes."

   d. "I've had this 'funny feeling' for a week."

   e. "I feel weak all over whenever I exert myself."

The Nursing Physical Assessment. As we have already discussed, physical assessment is performed in conjunction with the nursing interview. It is accomplished by means of a thorough, systematic examination of the patient. This examination includes the following activities:

☐ **Inspection:** Examination by careful and critical observation
☐ **Auscultation:** Examination by listening with a stethoscope
☐ **Palpation:** Examination by touching and feeling
☐ **Percussion:** Examination by touching, tapping, and listening

The actual skills of physical assessment (how to inspect, auscultate, percuss, and palpate) come with practice, and it is important to maintain an active use of these skills in order to maintain competency.

The method of organization that you choose to perform the physical exam will depend on your own preference and the condition of the patient. For example, many nurses use a "head-to-toe" method for the initial examination. If you choose to use the "head-to-toe" approach, you begin by assessing the head and neck (eyes, ears, nose, mouth, and throat). Then you continue down the body to the thorax, abdomen, legs, and feet, in that order. Other nurses prefer to use a "systems approach" to gathering data. They begin by assessing the respiratory system (nose, mouth, throat, lungs) and continue by assessing the cardiac status, the circulatory status, neurological status, gastrointestinal status, genitourinary status, musculoskeletal status, and status of the skin (integumentary system). The order in which you examine the patient will depend on his state of health. For example, if you have a well client, you may choose to begin wherever you would like, so long as you always use the same method. (Always using the same method lessens the likelihood of forgetting something.) On the other hand, if you have an ill patient, you should examine the area of the body where the problems are before you go onto the other parts of the body (*e.g.*, if the patient complains of abdominal discomfort, examine the abdomen first).

The following guidelines are suggested to help you when performing a physical assessment.

☐ *Guidelines*   *Performing a Physical Assessment*

☐ **Always Promote Communication** between yourself and the client. Introduce yourself, provide for privacy, establish rapport, and use good interviewing techniques while you are performing the physical assessment (rather than working in silence).

☐ **Don't Rely on Memory.** Jot down notes to be sure of accuracy.

☐ **Choose a Method of Organizing Your Assessment** and use it consistently. If you need a guide, use the method listed below, which prioritizes assessment.

a. **Respiratory status:** Airway, breath sounds, rate, depth, cough, symmetry, pain/discomfort

b. **Cardiac status:** Apical rate, rhythm, heart sounds, pain/discomfort

c. **Circulatory status:** Rate, rhythm, and quality of pulses (radial, brachial, carotid, femoral, dorsalis pedis), pain/discomfort

d. **Status of the skin:** Color, temperature, turgor, edema, lesions, hair distribution, pain/discomfort

e. **Neurological status:** Mental status; orientation; pupillary reaction; vision and appearance of the eyes; ability to hear, taste, feel, and smell; pain/discomfort

     f. Musculoskeletal status: Muscle tone, strength, gait, stability, range of motion, pain/discomfort

     g. Gastrointestinal status: Condition of the lips, tongue, gums, teeth; presence of gag reflex; presence of bowel sounds; presence of abdominal distention or tenderness; impaction; hemorrhoids; pain/discomfort.

     h. Genitourinary status: Presence of distended bladder, discharge (vaginal, uretheral), pain/discomfort

---

☐ *Practice Session*   *The Nursing Physical Assessment*
(Suggested Answers on page 167)

1. Since physical assessment and interviewing go hand in hand, use the following situations to practice focusing your interview questions upon areas of concern noted during the physical exam.

    a. You examine and find: The patient's hands and fingernails are filthy with ground-in dirt, although the rest of him is clean.

    You may state or ask:

    b. You examine and find: The patient has a lump on the back of his head.

    You may state or ask:

    c. You examine and find: The patient's respirations are 40.

    You may state or ask:

    d. You examine and find: The patient's right eye is red, teary, and inflamed.

    You may state or ask:

    e. You examine and find: The patient's teeth are discolored and full of caries.

    You may state or ask:

2. Now practice focusing your physical exam upon areas of concern voiced by the patient:

    a. Patient states: "I have had a rash that comes and goes."

    You may reply and examine:

    b. Patient states: "My stomach has been hurting me."

    You may reply and examine:

c. Patient states: "I find it burns when I urinate."

You may reply and examine:

d. Patient states: "I feel like I'm heavier than usual—like I'm bloated with fluid."

You may reply and examine:

e. Patient states: "I think I hurt my calf playing tennis."

You may reply and examine:

3. Practice prioritizing your order of physical assessment by listing at least two things that you would want to assess first when performing a nursing assessment for the case histories below.

Case History A

Chelsey DeMarino has been admitted with a medical diagnosis of gastroenteritis. You enter her room for the first time today. She is lying on her side holding a cold rag over her head. Her eyes are closed, and you notice that she appears somewhat flushed. There is an emesis basin nearby that is empty. Her emergency room record states that she is 28 years old, married, and a homemaker.

Case History B

You have been told that Mr. Daniels had his gallbladder removed two days ago. You go into his room, and he is sitting in a chair near his bed reading the newspaper. There are two unopened packs of cigarettes on his night stand. He has a heparin lock for antibiotics in his left arm. When you ask how he is, he replies, "OK . . . except I'm so sore I can't move too much . . . then I start to cough and that kills me."

Case History C

In a clinical conference, or with another student or nurse, choose a real patient, and discuss how you would organize your nursing assessment for that particular patient. That is, what would you assess first, and how would you proceed?

Identifying Subjective and Objective Data

When information is gathered during a nursing assessment, it is helpful to separate the information into two categories: subjective data and objective data. *Subjective data* are what the patient/client actually states (*e.g.*, "I'm tired."). These are his feelings and perceptions. *Objective data* are concrete, *observable* information such as vital signs, laboratory studies, and changes in physical appearance or behavior. The purpose of separating data into these two categories is to help you to compare what you observe to what the patient actually tells you. For example, if the patient states, "I feel like my heart is racing," and you observe that his pulse is 140 beats per minute, your observation verifies that what he *feels is* actually *happening.*

Sometimes you may find that what you observe and what the patient is stating are different. For example, the patient may state that he feels "okay," but you may note that his facial expression appears to be one of pain. This type of discrepancy between what you observe (objective data) and what the patient tells you (subjective data) often means that problem identification will be a little more difficult; it will take a bit more investigating to be sure that you have *all the pertinent information* necessary to understand the full scope of the problems.

You will find in Chapter 3 (where diagnosis is discussed) and Chapter 4 (where documentation is discussed) that knowing the difference between subjective and objective data is a key concept that you should understand. There is a trick for remembering these two categories of data:

S-S Subjective data are Stated.

O-O Objective data are Observable.

Note the examples of subjective and objective data listed below:

Subjective Data	Objective Data
"I feel sick to my stomach."	Blood pressure of 110/70
"I have a stabbing pain in my side."	Rash on right arm
	Walks with a limp
"I wish I were home."	Ate all of his breakfast
"I feel like nobody likes me."	Urinated 150 ml clear urine

☐ *Practice Session*   *Subjective and Objective Data*
(*Suggested Answers on page 168*)

Read the following case histories and answer the subsequent questions.

Case History A

Mr. Michaels is 51 years old. He was admitted two days ago with chest pain. His physician has ordered the following studies: electrocardiogram, chest x-ray, and complete blood studies including a blood sugar. These studies were just posted on the chart. When you talk with him, he states, "I feel much better today—no more pain. It is a relief to get rid of that discomfort." You think he appears a little tired or weary—he seems to be talking slowly and sighs more often than you would think is necessary. When his wife comes to see him, she is cheerful with him, but confides in you that he seems depressed or something. His vital signs are:

T: 98.6   P: 74 (regular)   R: 22   B/P: 140/90

1. List the subjective data noted in the case history given above (*i.e.*, what were you told directly?).

2. List the objective data noted in the case history given above (*i.e.*, what is Mr. Michaels's general behavior, and what information can be readily observed?).

Case History B

Mrs. Rochester is a 33-year-old mother of two young children. She is admitted with the medical diagnosis of diabetes. Today you enter her room, and she states, "The doctor says I have diabetes. I can't see how I could have diabetes. No one in my family has diabetes. I feel fine. . . . I don't see how I can make myself change the way I eat. Dieting drives me crazy. . . . That's why I weighed 190 pounds when you weighed me." On further questioning, she admits that she has been feeling unusually tired lately, and that she does seem to have to urinate more than usual. You check her chart and note that her fasting blood sugar was elevated at 144. Her vital signs are:

T: 98.1   P: 88 (regular)   R: 24   B/P: 144/88

1. List the subjective data noted in the case history given above (*i.e.*, what were you told directly?).

2. List the objective data noted in the case history given above (*i.e.*, what is Mrs. Rochester's general behavior, and what information can be readily observed?).

Case History C

In a clinical conference, or with another student or nurse, choose data from a real patient, and discuss and determine what are subjective data and what are objective data.

Identifying Cues and Making Inferences

The subjective and objective data that you identify act as cues. *Cues* are "hints" or "reminders" that prompt you to make a judgment or *inference*. Consider the following example:

You identify the following cues:

Subjective Data: Patient states "I just started taking penicillin for a tooth abscess"

Objective Data: Fine rash over trunk

The above data, when put together, give you *cues* that will probably lead you to *infer* that the person is having an allergic reaction to penicillin.

Inferences may be made about a single cue or a group of cues. But remember, the more cues you have, the more likely you are to make correct (valid) inferences. Your ability to identify *significant cues* and make *correct inferences* will be influenced by your observational skills, your nursing knowledge, and your expertise in clinical practice. Your *values and beliefs* will also influence how you interpret certain cues, so you must make a conscious effort to avoid making value judgments (*e.g.*, inferring that a person who bathes only once a week needs to be taught better hygiene, when actually this practice may be part of his culture).

To clarify your understanding of cues and inferences, study the examples of cues with corresponding inferences below.

Cue:	Judy states, "I have trouble moving my bowels."
Inference:	Judy may be constipated.
Cue:	Jeffrey is silent and withdrawn and has a sad face.
Inference:	Jeffrey may be depressed.
Cue:	Mrs. Rayburn's blood pressure is 60/50.
Inference:	Mrs. Rayburn is in shock.
Cue:	Susan states, "I can't stand this pain any more!"
Inference:	Susan is experiencing unbearable pain.

☐ *Practice Session*   *Identifying Cues and Making Inferences*
(Suggested Answers on page 168)

1. a. List the cues that you can identify in Case History A (Mr. Michaels, page 36).

    b. List the inferences that you might make about the cues that have been identified.

2. a. List the cues that you can identify in Case History B (Mrs. Rochester, page 37).

b. List the inferences that you might make about the cues that you have identified.

3. In a clinical conference (or with another student or nurse), choose data from a real patient, identify cues, and discuss the inferences you might make from the cues.

Validating Data

Data validation focuses upon making sure that your data are *factual*. This means that you have to be sure that the cues are correct and that your inferences, or interpretations, are correct. *If you are not sure about the validity of your information, you should obtain more data to verify what you have listed as facts, rather than go on to analyze and identify health problems,* because having incorrect information could cause you to make an error in problem identification.

Taking the time to gather more information to validate your data will help you to make sure that your information is factual and also *more complete*. This is because as you go through the process of verifying your data, you will often note additional information that has been overlooked. For example, because of a patient's withdrawn affect, you may have inferred that he is depressed. However, by saying, "Tell me how you're feeling," or "You seem very quiet—like you might be depressed," you gain more information that may validate what you have *inferred* (or further explain his withdrawn affect). By verifying your impressions, you have a clearer picture of the patient's health status, and you are more likely to be correct.

Validating data helps you to avoid:

☐ Missing pertinent information
☐ Misunderstanding situations
☐ Jumping to conclusions or focusing in the wrong direction

Experienced nurses are more adept at noting when information is questionable, or incomplete. However, if you are a beginner, you may want to have a more experienced nurse or faculty member assist you by checking your data (*i.e.*, validating your cues and/or inferences). The guidelines below are presented to help you learn or review methods of validating data.

□ Guidelines	*Validating Data*

□ Be aware that data that can be measured with an accurate scale of measurement can be accepted as factual (*e.g.*, a person who is measured to be 5 feet 6 inches and 145 pounds . . . a person who was born in 1935 . . . most laboratory studies).*

□ Keep in mind that data that someone else observes to be factual may or may not be true. When the information is critical, you should verify it by directly observing and interviewing the patient.

□ Form the habit of validating data that are questionable by using the following techniques, as appropriate:

Recheck Your Own Data (*e.g.*, take a blood pressure in the opposite arm or 10 minutes later)

Look for Temporary Factors That May Alter the Accuracy of Your Data (*e.g.*, check whether someone who has an elevated temperature and no other symptoms has just had a hot cup of tea)

Ask Someone Else, preferably an expert, to collect the same data (*e.g.*, ask a more experienced nurse to recheck a blood pressure when you're not sure)

Always Double-Check Data That Are Extremely Abnormal (*e.g.*, use two scales to check an infant who appears much heavier or lighter than the scale states)

Compare Your Subjective and Objective Data to see if what the patient is stating is congruent with what you observe (*e.g.*, compare actual pulse rate, with perceptions of "racing heart")

Clarify Patient and Family Statements and Verify Your Inferences (*e.g.*, say "to me, you seem tired")

□ Practice Session	*Validating Data*

(*Suggested Answers on page 169*)

1. a. From the cues and inferences that you identified in Case History A (Mr. Michaels, page 36), indicate in three separate columns those that you feel are *certainly valid, probably valid,* and only *possibly valid.*

---

* There is always the possibility of laboratory error or other factors that may alter the accuracy of the laboratory studies (*e.g.*, a fasting blood sugar that is done even though the person has eaten 1 hour before). Rechecking gross abnormalities should validate the studies.

b. For the data you list in the *possibly valid* and *probably valid* columns, identify some methods of clarifying if they are indeed true (*e.g.*, what other questions might you ask?).

2. a. From the cues and inferences that you identified in Case History B (Mrs. Rochester, page 37), indicate in three separate columns those that you feel are *certainly valid*, *probably valid*, and only *possibly valid*.

   b. For the data you list in the *possibly valid* and *probably valid* columns identify some methods of clarifying if they are indeed true (*e.g.*, what other questions might you ask?).

3. In a clinical conference, or with another student or nurse, choose data from a real patient, identify cues, and discuss the inferences you might make from the cues. Now discuss which cues and inferences are probably valid and what methods you might use for validation.

Organizing (Clustering) Data

After you have gathered and validated your patient's data, you will be ready to organize or cluster them into categories of information that will help you to identify patient strengths, and actual and potential health problems. How you organize the data will depend on your knowledge, skill, and preference. Often, experienced nurses will organize the data mentally, while newer nurses find it easier to organize the data on a separate piece of paper. As with the assessment tool for gathering data, many institutions and schools of nursing have a required or recommended method of organizing data. Maslow (Display 2-4), Gordon (Display 2-5), and the North American Nursing Diagnosis Association (Display 2-6) offer good methods of organizing data to maintain a *nursing focus.* This type of data organization will be very helpful when you identify nursing diagnoses because it brings related data together, and helps you to see patterns of human behavior.

To assist you in identifying problems that should be *referred* to the physician, the Body Systems approach (Display 2-7) will be helpful because

(*Text continues on page 44*)

Display 2-4. Clustering Assessment Data According to Human Needs (Maslow)

1. Cluster together data that pertain to physiological needs (survival needs).

   Examples: Food, fluids, oxygen, elimination, warmth, physical comfort

2. Cluster together data that pertain to safety and security needs.

   Examples: Those things necessary for physical safety (such as side rails on a bed) and psychological security (such as a child's favorite blanket)

3. Cluster together data that pertain to love and belonging needs.

   Example: Family members, significant others

4. Cluster together data that pertain to self-esteem needs.

   Example: Those things that make the individual feel good about himself (such as autonomy, independence)

5. Cluster together data that pertain to self-actualization needs.

   Example: The need to grow and change and accomplish goals

Display 2-5. Organization of Assessment Data According to Functional Health Patterns (Gordon)

1. *Health-perception–health-management pattern.* Describes client's perceived pattern of health and well-being and how health is managed

2. *Nutritional-metabolic pattern.* Describes pattern of food and fluid consumption relative to metabolic need and pattern indicators of local nutrient supply

3. *Elimination pattern.* Describes pattern of excretory function (bowel, bladder, and skin)

4. *Activity–exercise pattern.* Describes pattern of exercise, activity, leisure, and recreation

5. *Cognitive-perceptual pattern.* Describes sensory-perceptual and cognitive pattern

6. *Sleep-rest pattern.* Describes patterns of sleep, rest, and relaxation

7. *Self-perception–self-concept pattern.* Describes self-concept pattern and perceptions of self (e.g., body comfort, body image, feeling state)

8. *Role-relationship pattern.* Describes pattern of role-engagements and relationships

9. *Sexuality-reproductive pattern.* Describes client's patterns of satisfaction and dissatisfaction with sexuality pattern; describes reproductive patterns

10. *Coping-stress-tolerance pattern.* Describes general coping pattern and effectiveness of the pattern in terms of stress tolerance

11. *Value-belief pattern.* Describes patterns of values, beliefs (including spiritual), or goals that guide choices or decisions.

(Reproduced by permission from Gordon M: Nursing Diagnosis: Process and Application. New York, McGraw-Hill, 1982; copyrighted by the C.V. Mosby Co., St. Louis)

Display 2-6. Nine Human Response Patterns of the Unitary Person

1. *Exchanging:* A human response pattern involving mutual giving and receiving

2. *Communicating:* A human response pattern involving sending messages

3. *Relating:* A human response pattern involving establishing bonds

4. *Valuing:* A human response pattern involving the assigning of relative worth

5. *Choosing:* A human response pattern involving the selection of alternatives

6. *Moving:* A human response pattern involving activity

7. *Perceiving:* A human response pattern involving the reception of information

8. *Knowing:* A human response pattern involving the meaning associated with information

9. *Feeling:* A human response pattern involving the subjective awareness of information

(North American Nursing Diagnosis Association, St. Louis University School of Nursing, St. Louis, Missouri)

Display 2-7. Clustering Data According to Body Systems

(Helps to identify data that should be referred to the physician)

1. Cluster together a brief client profile (vital statistics), including the following:
   Name; age; reason the individual is seeking healthcare; vital signs; any known medical problems/diagnoses, allergies, or problems with diet.

2. Cluster together any data you suspect may be abnormal for any of the following systems:

   ☐ Respiratory system

   ☐ Cardiovascular system

   ☐ Nervous system

   ☐ Musculoskeletal system

   ☐ Gastrointestinal system

   ☐ Genitourinary system

   ☐ Integumentary system

physicians are involved in diagnosing abnormalities in systems or organ function. The diagram below shows the relationship between clustering data and identifying health problems.

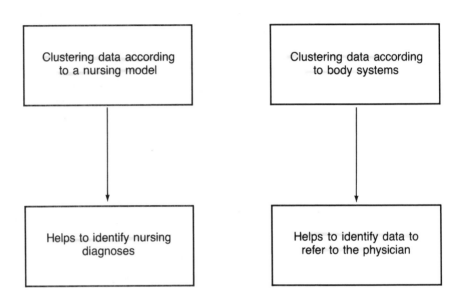

If you cluster data according to body systems only, you will be likely to be missing the key data that lead you to identifying nursing diagnoses. If you cluster data according to a nursing model, you should be sure that you are able to pull out and cluster together the data that are related to organ or system function. Having done this, you'll be better able to see problems with organ or system function (*i.e.*, problems that should be referred).

While the Functional Health Patterns and the Human Needs approaches offer good ways of clustering information to identify nursing diagnoses, and the Body Systems approach offers a good way to identify data that need to be referred to the physician, your school or hospital may recommend a different method. The key point is to find a good way of organizing data and to use it consistently, so that you gain expertise, and are systematic and comprehensive.

Display 2-8 shows the same patient data clustered according to Human Needs, Functional Health Patterns, and Body Systems.

Display 2-8. *Examples of the Same Patient Data Organized According to Human Needs, Functional Health Patterns, and Body Systems*

Data

1. 21-year-old male
2. Married, no children*
3. Occupation: Firefighter*
4. Ht: 6'1"; Wt: 170 lb
5. T: 98; P: 60; R: 16
6. B/P: 110/60
7. Unconscious from head injury
8. Spontaneous respirations
9. Lungs clear
10. History of seizures
11. Foley draining clear urine
12. Wife states he's always constipated
13. Tube feeding via nasogastric tube every 4 hours
14. Extremities rigid
15. Has reddened areas on both elbows
16. Allergic to penicillin
17. Wife states she feels as though she is falling apart*
18. Wife states that before the accident, he took pride in being physically fit*
19. Wife states that they were considering converting to Catholicism before the accident*

Data Organization by Maslow's Needs

Physical: 1, 4, 5, 6, 7, 8, 9, 10, 11, 12, 13, 14, 15, 16, 18

Safety/security: 7, 10, 13, 17, 19

Love and belonging: 2, 17, 19

Self-esteem: 2, 3, 18

Self-actualization: 3

Data Organization by Gordon's Functional Health Patterns

Health-perception–health-management pattern: 10, 18

Nutritional-metabolic pattern: 4, 5, 6, 8, 9, 11, 13, 15, 16

Elimination pattern: 11, 12, 13, 15

Activity-exercise pattern: 14

Cognitive-perceptual pattern: 7

Sleep-rest pattern: 7

Self-perception–self-concept pattern: 18

Role-relationship pattern: 1, 2, 3

Sexuality-reproductive pattern: 2

Coping-stress-tolerance pattern: 17

Value-belief pattern: 19

Data Organization by Body Systems to Determine What Should Be Referred to the Physician

Vital statistics (*client profile*): 1, 4, 5, 6, 7, 10, 16

Respiratory system: 8, 9

Cardiovascular system: 5, 6, 9

Nervous system: 7, 10

Musculoskeletal system: 14

Gastrointestinal system: 12, 13

Genitourinary system: 11

Integumentary system: 15

* These data are more likely to be clustered according to a nursing model only, and therefore are not assigned a category under the Body Systems Organization.

☐ *Practice Session*   *Organizing Assessment Data*
(Suggested Answers on page 169)

1. Using a separate sheet of paper, choose a method of organizing your data collection and organize the sets of data from the two case histories listed below.

   Case History A
   1. Age 20
   2. Single, lives with parents and two younger sisters
   3. Occupation: College student
   4. Religion: Protestant
   5. Medical diagnosis: Mononucleosis
   6. T: 101; P: 110; R: 30; B/P 110/84
   7. States he has a constant headache
   8. States he is depressed because he is missing school and is worried that his girlfriend may "catch mono too"
   9. Appetite poor
   10. He is weak when he stands or walks
   11. Before illness he was in good health and ran 5 miles a day
   12. Urine output in the past 16 hours is 250 ml
   13. Last bowel movement was 5 days ago—states he "can't stand using the portable commode"
   14. States he has a constant sore throat

   Case History B
   1. Age 36
   2. Married, has three small children
   3. Occupation: Landscape architect and homemaker
   4. Religion: Episcopalian
   5. Medical diagnosis: Pneumonia
   6. T: 100; P: 100; R: 28; B/P 104/68
   7. States she is concerned about how her husband is caring for the children—that it is "tough on him"
   8. States she feels weak and tired all the time, but can't seem to rest because she keeps coughing all the time.
   9. Appetite poor. Is forcing fluids well (1000 ml per shift)
   10. Before illness, she smoked a pack of cigarettes a day but has not smoked since hospitalization
   11. States she has always been in good health and has never had to be hospitalized (even gave birth at home)
   12. States all the tests that have to be done make her nervous—she is worried about getting AIDS from needle sticks
   13. Lungs have bilateral rhonchi. She coughs up thick yellow mucus
   14. Chest x-ray shows improvement over the past 2 days
   15. White blood cell count is elevated at 16,000

2. For each of the histories above, list the data that might signify or do signify a possible organ or system problem.

Identifying Patterns and Filling In the Gaps

Once you have clustered the data into groups of related information, you are ready for the final phase of assessment: identifying patterns and filling in the gaps of missing data. Using the puzzle analogy, you examine many pieces of information and put some of the pieces of the picture together. Because you have quite a few of the pieces together, you can now more readily identify key missing pieces. (How much easier it is to find key pieces as you near completion of the puzzle!) You begin to get some initial impressions about the presence of certain patterns as you study the data that you have clustered together. These initial impressions are often helpful in guiding you to identify gaps in data collection. Consider the following example in which a nurse has used a Human Needs approach and clustered the data under safety and security needs:

☐ Is a 72-year-old male

☐ Is blind

☐ States that he's always hurting himself

☐ States that he uses a cane to detect objects in front of him

☐ Has visible bumps and bruises over arms and on head

This information may suggest to you that this individual has a potential for injury. However, there is not enough data to determine *why* he has a potential for injury. Is it only because he is blind? Perhaps he is falling down because of weakness or dizziness. After all, if he's using the cane correctly, do you think he would be bumping himself all the time? These questions and thoughts that come to mind while you are gathering and clustering data should guide you to gather additional information to describe the problems more clearly. For example, with the above patient, you would need to use probing questions and ask the person to clarify *how* and *why* he keeps hurting himself. You may find that he is hurting himself because he is fainting, or does not use the cane properly, or is a victim of abuse. All of these questions can only be answered by filling in the gaps in information that you originally gathered. In other words, part of identifying patterns involves making an initial impression, noting gaps in the data you have gathered, and probing to fill in those gaps.

Just as with clustering data and validating data, your ability to identify patterns and focus data collection to fill in gaps of information will grow with your nursing knowledge and skill. You will get better at focusing your assessment once a possible problem emerges (asking the right questions and examining the right parts). You will learn to identify patterns of health and illness, and to be more complete. What is important to remember is that the extra time you take now to fill in gaps in data collection will be invaluable when you go on to the next steps of the nursing process, when you actually identify the health problems and set forth a plan of care. By being comprehensive, you will be *less* likely to:

☐ Miss problems

☐ Identify problems that are not there

☐ Mislabel problems

☐ Identify interventions that are not likely to work

You will be *more* likely to:

☐ Identify client strengths

☐ Identify all the problems

☐ Label the problems correctly

☐ Identify appropriate individualized interventions

Communicating/Recording Data

Verbal communication of significant findings (*e.g.*, abnormal vital signs, pain, problems with breathing or circulation) should be given priority over completing nursing data base records. That is, whenever you have identified data that you suspect may be indicative of a problem that requires the attention of a more qualified professional (*e.g.*, primary nurse, head nurse, physician), you should report the information as soon as possible. Reporting significant data expedites interventions that are beyond your expertise, and alerts the key people involved that their presence may be required.

Having communicated significant data to the appropriate individuals, you are now ready to complete the nursing data base record. Almost every facility has a required data base assessment form that must be completed. However, if you are not required to complete a specific form, you should record your findings according to the following guidelines.

☐ *Guidelines*   *Recording the Nursing Data Base*

☐ Use ink, and write or print legibly.

☐ Follow precisely hospital/facility/school policies and procedures for recording the data base.

☐ Follow an organized method of recording data (*e.g.*, the data base on page 17 or 22).

□ Document the name of any person contributing to the history other than the patient.

□ Be clear when you record what you observed.

> *Right:* Breath sounds diminished at left lower base, and he complains of piercing pain upon inspiration.
>
> *Wrong:* Seems to be having difficulty breathing.

□ Write patient statements using the patient's own words (*e.g.*, "it feels like a knife's cutting me in two when I move the wrong way").

□ Chart whom you notified if you have reported significant data.

□ Chart the most critical data first (*e.g.*, vital signs, medications, allergies), so that if you leave the unit for some reason, they will be readily available.

Having reported significant data, and completed and recorded a comprehensive nursing assessment (*yet being fully aware that assessment continues whenever you interact with the patient*), you are now ready to go onto the next step of the nursing process: diagnosis.

KEY POINTS Assessment

1. *Assessment* is the first step of the nursing process when client information is gathered and examined in preparation for the second step: *Diagnosis*.

2. Although the primary source of information is the patient, comprehensive data collection includes gathering information from the following resources: families, significant others, nursing and medical records, verbal and written consultations with other health-care professionals, and relevant literature.

3. Identification of nursing diagnoses requires the comprehensive, *holistic data collection* that provides information about both the medical problems and how the person lives his daily life as a biopsychosocial human being.

4. Your ability to identify health problems depends on your skill in performing a *data base assessment* and a *focus assessment*.

5. *Subjective* data (gathered by use of interviewing techniques) and *objective data* (gathered by physical examination techniques) complement and clarify one another.

6. Subjective and objective data are *cues* (hints or reminders) that lead you to make an *inference* or judgment about what the data mean.

7. Your ability to identify cues and to make an inference about their significance will depend upon your assessment skills, knowledge of theory, and clinical expertise.

8. Validating data helps to ensure that your information is *factual* and *complete*.

9. Clustering related data together helps you to identify patterns, missing pieces of information, and (ultimately) client strengths and problems.

(Continued)

10. Clustering data according to a *nursing model* will assist to identify *nursing diagnoses*, while clustering data according to *body systems* will assist you to identify data that should be *referred* to the physician.

11. If you cluster data according to body systems only, then it would be as if you only put together selected pieces of the puzzle: only half your work is done, and you will be likely to be missing the key data that lead you to identifying nursing diagnoses.

Bibliography

American Nurses' Association (1973) *Standards of Nursing Practice.* Kansas City, MO.

Aspinall, M. and Tanner, C. (1985) *Decision-Making for Patient Care, Applying the Nursing Process.* Norwalk, CT: Appleton-Lange.

Bates, B. (1986) *A Guide to Physical Examination.* 3rd ed. Philadelphia: JB Lippincott.

Bellack, J. and Bamford, P. (1984) *Nursing Assessment: A Multidimensional Approach.* Montery, CA: Wadsworth Health Science Division.

Carnevali, D. (1984) *Nursing Care Planning: Diagnosis and Management.* Philadelphia: JB Lippincott.

Carnevali, D., Mitchell, P., Woods, N., and Tanner, C. (1984) *Diagnostic Reasoning in Nursing.* Philadelphia: JB Lippincott.

Carpenito, L. (1987) *Nursing Diagnosis: Application to Clinical Practice.* 2nd ed. Philadelphia: JB Lippincott.

Carpenito, L. (1987) *Handbook of Nursing Diagnosis.* 2nd ed. Philadelphia: JB Lippincott.

Chrisman, M. and Fowler, M. (1980) The systems-in-change model for nursing practice. In Riehl, J., and Royc, C. (eds.): *Conceptual Models for Nursing Practice.* Norwalk, CT: Appleton-Lange.

Dossy, B. (1979) Perfecting your skill in systematic patient assessments. *Nursing* 9:42–45.

Gordon, M. (1982) *Nursing Diagnosis: Process and Application.* New York: McGraw-Hill.

Griffith, J. and Christensen, P. (1982) *Nursing Process: Application of Theories, Frameworks and Models.* St. Louis: CV Mosby.

Guzzetta, K., Bunton, S., Prinkey, L., Sherer, A., and Seifert, P. (1988) Unitary person assessment tool: Easing the problems with nursing diagnoses. *Focus* 15(2):12–24.

King, I. (1971) *Toward a Theory of Nursing.* Boston: Little, Brown & Co.

Maslow, A. (1970) *Motivation in Personality.* New York: Harper & Row.

Orem, D. (1980) *Nursing: Concepts of Practice.* 2nd ed. New York: McGraw-Hill.

Rogers, M. (1969) *Introduction to the Thoretical Basis of Nursing.* New York: FA Davis.

Roy, C. (1976) *Introduction to Nursing: An Adaptation Model.* Englewood Cliffs: Prentice–Hall.

Soares, C. (1978) Nursing and medical diagnoses: A comparison of variant and essential features. In Chaska, N. (ed.): *The Nursing Profession: Views Through the Mist.* New York: McGraw-Hill.

Vaughan-Wroble, B. and Perkins, S. (1986) Nursing diagnoses: The pivotal point of the nursing process in cardiovascular nursing. *Cardiovascular Nursing* (22)5:25-29.

Yura, H. and Walsh, M.B. (1988) *The Nursing Process.* 5th ed. Norwalk, CT: Appleton-Lange.

Ziegler, S., Vaughan-Wroble, B., and Erlen, J. (1986) Nursing Process, Nursing Diagnosis, Nursing Knowledge: Avenues to Autonomy. Norwalk, CT: Appleton-Lange.

☑ Analyzing Data
☑ Identifying Nursing Diagnoses
☑ Identifying Collaborative Problems
☑ Identifying Strengths

3
Diagnosis

Standard II: *Nursing diagnoses are derived from health-status data.**

*Abstracted from Standards of Nursing Practice. Copyright American Nurses' Association, 1973

Glossary

Category Label A title that gives a concise description of a nursing diagnosis.

Collaborative Problem An actual or potential health problem (complication) that focuses upon the *pathophysiologic response* of the body (to trauma, disease, diagnostic studies, or treatment modalities) and that nurses are responsible and accountable for identifying and treating *in collaboration with the physician.*

Defining Characteristics A cluster of signs, symptoms, and risk factors often seen with a certain nursing diagnosis.

Diagnostic Error When a health problem has been overlooked or incorrectly identified.

Diagnostic Reasoning A method of thinking that involves specific, deliberate use of logic to reach conclusions about an individual's health state.

Diagnostic Statement A phrase that clearly describes a health problem.

Etiology The cause or contributing factors of a health problem (see also, **Risk Factor**).

Independent Nursing Intervention An action prescribed and performed by a nurse that requires no written protocol or physician's order.

Intuition Knowing something without supporting evidence.

Medical Diagnosis A traumatic or disease condition which is validated by medical diagnostic studies, and for which treatment focuses upon correction or preventing *pathology of specific organs or body systems* (requires treatment by a licensed physician).

NANDA Acronym for the North American Nursing Diagnosis Association.

Nursing Diagnosis An actual or potential health problem that focuses upon the *holistic (human) response* of an individual or group, and that nurses are responsible and accountable for identifying and treating *independently.*

Possible Nursing Diagnosis A nursing diagnosis that may or may not be present as evidenced by some ambiguous cues in the assessment data. The ambiguous cues direct the nurse to gather more data to clarify what the cues mean and to confirm whether the defining characteristics for that diagnostic category are indeed present.

Potential Nursing Diagnosis A nursing diagnosis for which a person is at risk as evidenced by the presence of risk factors noted during the nursing assessment.

Qualification Having the knowledge and authority to do something.

Risk Factor Something known to contribute to or create a specific problem (see also, **Etiology**).

Sign   An objective manifestation of a health problem.

Symptom   A subjective manifestation of a health problem.

Wellness   A state of optimal biopsychosocial functioning.

Diagnosis: Identifying Strengths and Problems

During assessment, you have gathered and examined data, and you've begun to note patterns of health and illness. Now, during this step, *diagnosis*, you will finish "putting it all together" to identify the problems (which will be the basis of the care plan) and strengths (which will be used and reinforced to develop an efficient and effective plan of care). This chapter will discuss the evolution of nursing diagnosis, give guidelines for diagnostic reasoning (how to identify individual problems and strengths by using both logic and intuition), and provide the "how to's" of recognizing and stating nursing diagnoses and other health problems.

The Evolution of Nursing Diagnosis

During the past two decades, nursing has experienced a 180° turn in both responsibilities and focus. Before the 1970s, nurses were responsible for *assessing* patients, but were not allowed to make *judgments* about their observations. The responsibility of making diagnoses was limited by law to physicians. Nursing education focused more upon teaching nurses to assist physicians to treat diseases than to act independently to treat unique human responses. However, in time, the role of the nurse began to expand, and the American Nurses Association (ANA) recognized a need to publish new standards for nursing practice that included the role of the nurse as a diagnostician (*ANA Standards of Nursing Practice*, 1973). These standards were followed by the publication of the ANA *Social Policy Statement* (1980), which stated that "nursing is the diagnosis and treatment of human responses to actual and potential health problems." With these publications (and with subsequent changes in nurse practice acts), nurses became responsible and accountable for making *nursing diagnoses*, and their focus became one of *treating the whole person*, not just the disease.

Because of these changes, nursing has had to look for answers to some tough questions: How does nursing diagnosis differ from medical diagnosis? What is a human response? Is it how the individual feels he is reacting to an actual or potential health problem, how it is causing difficulty with daily living? Or can it include, for example, how his liver responds? Do nursing diagnoses include pathophysiologic responses? Healthy responses? How does a nurse assess and intervene for a nursing diagnosis? Nurses were challenged to find answers.

To meet this challenge and to identify categories of problems that should be considered to be nursing diagnoses, a group of nurses (made up of theorists, educators, administrators, and practitioners) met in 1973 to form the National Conference Group for the Classification of Nursing Diagnoses. As a result of their work, a list of diagnoses that were accepted for study and clinical testing was developed (1973). This group has since become the North American Nursing Diagnosis Association (NANDA) and has held national meetings every two years. At these meetings, the ongoing work of its committee members is discussed, the membership has the opportunity to exchange ideas and concerns (both formally and informally), relevant continuing education programs are offered, and newly submitted nursing diagnoses are presented to the membership. After discussion at the meeting, the members vote whether to accept each diagnosis for study. The NANDA list, updated in 1988, appears on the inside cover of this book, and is addressed in more depth in the *Nursing Diagnosis Quick Reference Section* beginning on page 181. While NANDA is clear that the list needs further study, it has been widely accepted for use in identifying nursing diagnoses.

We have made great strides in the evolution of nursing diagnoses. However, because we are *still evolving*, and will continue to evolve, you will find varied views on how nursing diagnoses should be defined, whether they should describe both healthy and unhealthy responses, and exactly how nurses should intervene once they've diagnosed that a health problem exists. There is, however, a consensus that nurses indeed do diagnose: They perform an assessment, examine and study the data (*analyze* the information), and pull it together (*synthesize* the information) to make diagnoses concerning the patient's health status.

The diagram below illustrates how the steps of assessment lead to diagnosis.

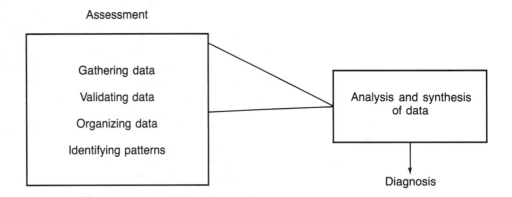

Let's take a look at the process of diagnostic reasoning, that is, *how to analyze and synthesize data* to make a diagnosis of health or illness.

Diagnostic Reasoning

The process of analyzing data and pulling it together to make a diagnosis, or a method of thinking that uses logic to come to conclusions about an individual's health status, is called *diagnostic reasoning*. Your ability to identify nursing diagnoses and other health problems with accuracy will depend upon your ability to be methodical, systematic, and logical in coming to conclusions about your patient's problems and strengths.

The following presents *fundamental principles* and *suggested steps* for diagnostic reasoning. These principles can be applied to diagnosing all health problems (both nursing diagnoses and problems that should be referred to the physician).

Fundamental Principles of Diagnostic Reasoning

The following are fundamental principles of diagnostic reasoning.

☐ Problem identification begins with asking the patient (and family) to describe anything that seems to be causing problems. For example: "Can you think of anything happening in your life that could be, or has been affecting your health?"

Rationale: Often it will be the patient and his family who will best be able to efficiently identify any problems.

☐ Your ability to be proficient at diagnosing health problems and strengths is dependent upon your knowledge of nursing and your clinical expertise. Display 3-1 lists categories of nursing knowledge.

Display 3-1. Nursing Knowledge

The greater your depth of knowledge in the following areas, the more likely you are to be a good diagnostician.

Health promotion	Practice wisdom*
Growth and development	Anatomy and physiology
Mental health/psychiatry	Disease process/treatment
Community health/group dynamics	Diagnostic/monitoring modalities
Culture/ethics/law	Pathophysiology/pharmacology
Research/leadership	Microbiology/chemistry
Teaching/communication	Physical and social sciences
Technical skills	

Practice wisdom is a term coined by Ziegler and Vaughn-Wrobel in 1986 to include knowledge of tradition, ethics, authority, and trial and error. I have added intuition, logic, and setting priorities.

Rationale: Making diagnoses often involves application of all of the categories of knowledge listed in Display 3-1. As your knowledge in all of these categories grows, so will your ability to be a good diagnostician.

☐ Students and nurses must be aware of their qualifications *and* limitations.

Rationale: An individual who enters the healthcare system has the right to be assessed by a *qualified* healthcare professional and to be informed when actual and potential health problems are identified. While you may feel that you have the knowledge to perform an assessment and diagnose the problems, you must determine (for your patient's health and your own legal protection) whether you are *authorized* to perform the assessment. Authority to perform assessments is derived from the following:

Laws/licensure/certification

National/state/community standards

Institutional standards/policies/procedures/protocols

Instructors/supervisors/physicians/schools of nursing

☐ Students and nurses who doubt their qualifications (whether they have the knowledge and authority) to perform an assessment or make diagnoses, must consult with an *appropriate resource* (*e.g.*, instructor, more qualified nurse, physician, dietician, pharmacist, text, policy manual).

Rationale: The responsibility of the diagnostician includes consulting with more qualified professionals and appropriate literature to assure a *safe and expedient* diagnosis.

☐ Before you can expect to identify *abnormal data,* you will have to be able to recognize *normal data.* For example, you won't recognize abnormal vital signs until you know normal variations in vital signs.

Rationale: Abnormalities are identified by comparing what is considered to be normal data with your patient's data. If there is a significant discrepancy, then you have identified an abnormality, which may indicate a problem. Display 3-2 gives guidelines for identifying abnormal data.

☐ Beginning diagnosticians must understand the terms *sign, symptom, defining characteristics,* and *cues.* (See Display 3-3 for clarification of these terms.)

Rationale: Signs, symptoms, and defining characteristics are like the *key pieces of the puzzle:* If you do not have them, you cannot "complete the puzzle" and label the problem.

☐ If you do not have a mental storehouse of the names, definitions, defining characteristics (or common signs and symptoms) and common causes of

Display 3-2. Questions to Ask to Determine Normal and Abnormal

Ask the Person:

☐ Would you say this is normal or abnormal for you?

☐ What would you describe as normal for you?

Ask Yourself:

☐ Is what the individual accepts as "normal" detrimental to his health?

☐ What is "normal" for a person who is this individual's age and physical stature?

☐ What is "normal" for a person who has this individual's type of beliefs or culture?

☐ What is "normal" for a person who has this occupation, this socioeconomic level, these favorite activities, this lifestyle?

☐ Do today's data, when compared to the data collected before intervention began (baseline data), show abnormalities?

☐ What is "normal" for a person with this disease process?

☐ Are there too many "slightly abnormal" factors that, when put together, may signify an overall picture of abnormality?

Display 3-3. Definitions of Diagnostic Terms

Sign: *Objective data** that has been *known to signify* a health problem (*e.g.*, fever is a sign).

Symptom: *Subjective data** that has been *known to signify* a health problem (*e.g.*, pain is a symptom).

Defining Characteristics: Clusters of signs, symptoms, and risk factors that are observed in a patient with a specific nursing diagnosis.

Cues: All data that prompt you to suspect a health problem (*i.e.*, the presence of defining characteristics, signs, and symptoms).

*Often the terms objective and subjective data are used interchangeably with signs and symptoms. However, technically, objective data include all the data that you observe (normal and abnormal), and subjective data include all the data that the patient tells you (normal and abnormal).

health problems, you should carry with you a reference or references that can provide this information for you.

Rationale: You cannot expect to identify health problems if you do not know what they look like. By carrying this type of reference with you, you can diagnose problems by comparing your patient's data with the data presented in the reference.

☐ Nurses and students must be aware that if they miss a problem, mislabel a problem, or identify a problem that is not there, this is a *diagnostic error,* which can result in *inappropriate treatment.*

Rationale: An error in diagnosis is likely to cause an error in treatment because you will plan nursing actions *based upon the diagnoses or problems* that you have identified. Display 3-4 lists the possible consequences of making a diagnostic error.

Display 3-4. **Risks of Diagnostic Errors**

When you miss a problem, mislabel a problem, or fail to fully understand a problem, you run the risk of any of the following:

☐ Initiating interventions that actually aggravate the problems.

☐ Omitting interventions that are essential to solving the problems.

☐ Allowing problems to exist or progress without even detecting they are there.

☐ Initiating interventions that are harmless, but wasteful of everyone's time and energy.

☐ Influencing others that problems exist as described incorrectly.

☐ Placing yourself in danger of legal liability.

☐ Intuition can be used to expedite problem identification, as long as you follow the guidelines listed in Display 3-5, which describe how to use intuition safely.

Rationale: Intuition can be valuable in expediting problem identification, and knowing how to act safely on feelings of intuition will help you to act in the patient's best interest.

Display 3-5. Guidelines for Using the Nursing Process to Act Safely Upon Intuitive Feelings

☐ Acknowledge that your intuition is working, that you have no "hard data" to substantiate your feelings that a specific problem exists.

☐ Recognize that your intuition is sending up a "red flag" that says, "There is a problem here— watch this patient closely," or "This patient needs help." Assess closely for existing signs and symptoms that validate the presence of the problem that you suspect. (You should say to the patient, physician, or another nurse, "My intuition tells me that . . . " or "I have the feeling that . . . .")

☐ If you know that something is wrong, but can't put your finger on any specific problem, increase the frequency and intensity of nursing assessment to monitor closely for early detection of signs and symptoms.

☐ Before you act on intuition alone, weigh the risks of the possibility of your actions harming the patient (either aggravating the situation or creating new problems) against the risk of not acting at all (other than to actively monitor more closely).

Suggested Steps for Diagnostic Reasoning

The following steps are suggested to guide the process of diagnostic reasoning:

Step #1.   After you have completed data collection, study the information and *bring together related cues* (*e.g.*, signs and symptoms that relate to problems with safety, signs and symptoms that relate to problems with elimination).

Rationale: Bringing together related cues helps you to begin to get a picture of the problem.

Step #2.   If you identify one sign or symptom, or significant historical fact, focus your assessment to *look for additional signs, symptoms, or contributing history* that are often associated with the sign, symptom, or history. For example, if you identify a fever, look for signs and symptoms of infection (*i.e.*, pain, redness, swelling, heat, drainage, productive cough, history of contact with a communicable disease).

Rationale: Sometimes you will have a piece of data that you recognize as a sign or symptom, but you may not be able to determine its exact significance (*i.e.*, you do not have enough information to be sure). By using techniques of *focus assessment* to gather more information to determine whether other data that are often associated with that particular sign or symptom are present, you will be better able to pinpoint the problem.

Step #3.   Use a checklist to prompt you to check for common problems that are often encountered. (For example, see Display 3-6.)

Rationale: Using a checklist helps you to be both systematic and comprehensive in focusing your assessment and considering the types of problems that you should be looking for.

Step #4.   Form the habit of trying to think of more than one possible problem that the patient's cues could represent. For example, if your data suggest that your patient may be angry, consider *another explanation* for your patient's behavior. Is it possible that he is afraid?

Rationale: If you consider several problems that data could indicate, you will be less likely to come to a premature conclusion and make a diagnostic error.

Step #5.   Once you have listed the suspected problems, compare your patient's data with the defining characteristics (signs and symptoms or risk factors) that you have listed. Name the problem by using the label that most closely resembles your patient's data. For example, if you suspect that the patient has the nursing diagnosis of either anxiety or fear, compare your patient's data with the defining characteristics of anxiety and fear. If the data are most similar to anxiety, label the problem anxiety. If the data are most similar to the defining characteristics of fear, label the problem fear.

Rationale: Diagnosis is based upon recognizing that your patient's data contain the defining characteristics or signs and symptoms of a given problem.

Display 3-6. Checklist for Identifying Problem Areas

(circle one)

Are there pre-existing medical problems (disease/trauma)?	Yes	No	Pot*	Pos**
Are there pre-existing nursing problems (problems with activities of daily living)?	Yes	No	Pot	Pos
Is there a problem with breathing or circulation?	Yes	No	Pot	Pos
Is there a problem with nutrition or elimination?	Yes	No	Pot	Pos
Is there a problem with fluid intake/output?	Yes	No	Pot	Pos
Is there a problem with safety (risk for injury)?	Yes	No	Pot	Pos
Is there a problem with rest or exercise?	Yes	No	Pot	Pos
Is there a problem with ability to think or perceive environment?	Yes	No	Pot	Pos
Is there a problem with communication?	Yes	No	Pot	Pos
Is there a problem with role/relationships/sexuality?	Yes	No	Pot	Pos
Is there high risk for infection transmission?	Yes	No	Pot	Pos
Is there high risk for impairment of skin integrity?	Yes	No	Pot	Pos
Is this admission going to cause difficulties at home?	Yes	No	Pot	Pos
Is there a problem with coping or stress?	Yes	No	Pot	Pos
Is there a psychological/developmental/sociocultural problem?	Yes	No	Pot	Pos
Is there a problem with personal/religious beliefs?	Yes	No	Pot	Pos
Is there a problem with health maintenance at home?	Yes	No	Pot	Pos
Does the person have a problem with taking medications?	Yes	No	Pot	Pos
Does the patient require teaching?	Yes	No	Pot	Pos

*Pot = Potential problem (data demonstrates *no signs and symptoms* of the problem, but does demonstrate *risk factors* for the problem)

**Pos = Possible problem (data are vague, but examiner suspects that the problem may exist)

Step #6. Once you have identified problems, attempt to determine the cause or contributing factors of the problem.

Rationale: Sometimes you might not see the *main* problem at first. For example, you might assess a newly diagnosed diabetic patient and suspect that he has a problem with motivation to learn about insulin. If you delve further to determine what is causing this lack of motivation, you may find that the client is denying his disease. This problem of denial is the main problem now. Once you have dealt with that problem, you will be able to begin patient teaching.

Step #7. When possible, state both the problem and its etiology (cause or contributing factors), using the words "related to" to link the problem with its etiology. If you do not know the etiology, simply state the problem, and add "related to unknown factors" or "possibly related to . . . ."

Rationale: If you can describe both the problem and its cause, you can more readily identify actions for treatment. For example, compare the two problems below and note how *a* directs interventions while *b* provides little help.

a. *Ineffective Airway Clearance related to incisional pain and fear of splitting incision*

b. *Ineffective Airway Clearance*

Step # 8.   If your data demonstrate risk factors for a problem, but there are no signs and symptoms for the problem, then label it a *potential problem* and list the problem and contributing factors, using related to (*e.g., Potential Impaired Skin Integrity related to bedrest*).

Rationale: Labeling potential problems and identifying risk factors assists nurses to implement a plan to prevent problems *before* they occur.

Step #9.   If you suspect a problem, but do not have data to confirm the diagnosis, label it a *possible problem,* and continue to collect data to determine whether the problem exists (*e.g., Possible Self-Esteem Disturbance*).

Rationale: Listing possible problems alerts other nurses to monitor the patient for the suspected problem.

Suggested Steps for Identifying Strengths

The previous section guides you in the use of diagnostic reasoning to identify *problems.* But, since nurses must also be able to identify *patient strengths,* the following steps are suggested to assist you to diagnose strengths:

Step #1. Start by asking the individual (and family), "Can you tell me some things about yourself that you view as strengths, as healthy aspects?"

Rationale: Answers to this question will help you to identify strengths and helps the individual (and family) to recognize assets.

Step #2.   Study the patient's normal data, apply your knowledge of health, and tell the patient (and family) that these normal findings indicate healthy functioning in that specific area. For example, you might say, "You've made the decision to seek help, which is a healthy thing to do."

Rationale: This helps both you and the patient to focus on strengths as well as problems.

Step #3.   Together with the patient (and family), list the strengths that will assist you in preventing, resolving, or controlling the problems that you have identified. (For examples, see Display 3-7.)

Rationale: These are the strengths that you should use to develop an efficient care plan.

Display 3-7. Examples of Client Strengths

Physical Strengths

☐ Is in good health: exercises daily and has excellent cardiac and respiratory reserve

☐ Is in good nutritional state: eats three balanced meals with few snacks

☐ Demonstrates physical adaptation: upper torso and arms are powerful (compensating for para-plegia)

Psychological/Personal Strengths

☐ Demonstrates effect coping: states she copes with chronic pain by using guided imagery

☐ Is motivated: states he wants to learn about diabetes because he wants to be independent and healthy

☐ Verbalizes spiritual peace: priest brings daily communion

☐ Is knowledgeable: relates healthcare management and available resources

☐ Demonstrates good problem-solving skills: able to adjust daughter's therapy schedule for optimum results and convenience

☐ Has strong support systems: mother, brother, church are available for help with child care

☐ Utilizes personal/family resources: states she will ask daughter and best friend for rides to therapy

☐ Utilizes community resources: church, "meals on wheels"

☐ Positive healthcare management: demonstrates effective self-regulation of diet and insulin doses

---

☐ *Practice Session*   *Using Diagnostic Reasoning to Identify Signs and Symptoms*
(*Suggested Answers on p. 170*)

Practice identifying *normal* and *abnormal*, and *signs* and *symptoms*, by completing the two exercises below.

1. Study the objective and subjective data below. In the first space to the right, put "*nl*" next to the *normal data, abnl* next to the *abnormal data*.

   a. States he's been feeling fine.   ____ ____

   b. Temperature of 101°F.   ____ ____

   c. Pulse rate of 72 and regular (adult).   ____ ____

   d. Pulse rate of 150 (adult).   ____ ____

   e. Has hives over entire body.   ____ ____

   f. Infant cries as mother leaves the room.   ____ ____

   g. Patient complains of pain with urination.   ____ ____

    h. Grandmother suddenly does not recognize   ____   ____
        favorite grandchild.

    i. Grandmother says, "I can see okay   ____   ____
       as long as I wear my glasses."

    j. Infant cries, pulls at ears, and cannot   ____   ____
       be consoled by his mother.

2. Go back to exercise above. In the second space to the right, place "si" if it is a sign, "sy" if it is a symptom, "0" if it is *neither* a sign nor a symptom.

Nursing Diagnoses vs. Collaborative Problems

Now that we have examined the process of making a diagnosis, let's take a look at how nursing diagnosis differs from other health problems.

Gordon describes a nursing diagnosis as an "actual or potential health problem that nurses, by virtue of their education and experience, are capable and licensed to treat" (Gordon, 1976). Moritz states that nursing diagnoses are "responses to actual or potential health problems which nurses by virtue of their education and experience are able, licensed, and legally responsible and accountable to treat" (Moritz, 1984). Carpenito (1987) states that every problem that a nurse identifies is not necessarily a nursing diagnosis. She believes that nurses are involved in identifying two types of problems: *nursing diagnoses* (which involve the *independent role* of the nurse) and *collaborative problems* (which involve the *collaborative or interdependent role* of the nurse). Here is how she defines these two types of problems:

> *Nursing diagnosis:* A statement that describes the human response (health state or actual/potential altered interaction pattern) of an individual or group that the nurse can legally identify and for which the nurse can order definitive interventions to maintain the health state or to reduce, eliminate, or prevent alterations.

> *Collaborative problem:* A physiological complication that has resulted or may result from pathophysiological and treatment-related situations. Nurses monitor to detect their onset/status and collaborate with medicine for definitive treatment.

Carpenito's idea of using different terms (*nursing diagnosis* and *collaborative problem*) for the two types of problems that nurses treat has great merit. She points out that if we label all of the problems nurses identify as *nursing diagnoses*, we may be forcing nurses to make choices that are not in the patient's best interest and legally hazardous to the nurse. For example, suppose a nurse identifies the signs and symptoms of congestive heart failure and labels it a nursing diagnosis? If the nurse does not recognize that this problem belongs to medicine, might she not delay in referring the problem? And might not a court of law suggest that this nurse is practicing medicine (*i.e.*, making a medical diagnosis of congestive heart failure)?

Using two different terms to describe the types of problems that nurses identify helps us to examine both the *independent* and the *interdependent* or collaborative roles of the nurse. In this book, the terms *nursing diagnosis* and *collaborative problem* will be defined as follows:

> **Nursing Diagnosis:** An actual or potential health problem that focuses upon the *human response* of an individual or group, and that nurses are responsible and accountable for identifying and treating *independently.*

> **Collaborative Problem:** An actual or potential health problem (complication) that focuses upon the *pathophysiologic response* of the body (to trauma, disease, diagnostic studies, or treatment modalities), and that nurses are responsible and accountable to identify and treat *in collaboration with the physician.*

The diagram below illustrates the key question you must ask to determine whether you have identified a nursing diagnosis or a collaborative problem.

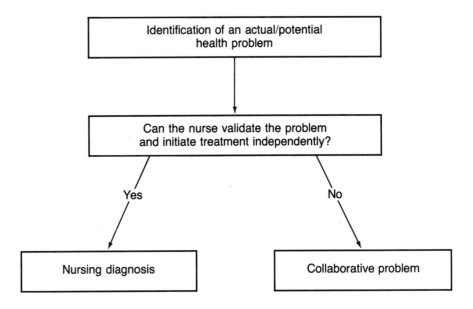

If you consider the definition of collaborative problem above, you may note a similarity to the definition of *medical diagnosis* below:

> **Medical Diagnosis:** A traumatic or disease condition that is validated by medical diagnostic studies, and for which treatment focuses upon correcting or preventing *pathology of specific organs or body systems* (requires treatment by a licensed physician).

Because both medical diagnoses and collaborative problems focus upon pathology or pathophysiology of organs or systems, *all medical diagnoses are collaborative problems.* For example, if your patient has a medical diagnosis of myocardial infarction, you would have to identify the *potential complications* associated with myocardial infarction (*e.g.,* arrhythmias, congestive heart failure).

While all medical diagnoses are collaborative problems for the nurse, not all collaborative problems are medical diagnoses. For example, chest tubes, nasogastric tubes, and intravenous lines are all considered collaborative problems, but are not medical diagnoses.

Table 3-1 compares the assessment focus, method of problem identification, and treatments in nursing diagnoses with those for collaborative problems and medical diagnoses.

Table 3-1. *Comparison of Nursing Diagnoses with Collaborative Problems and Medical Diagnoses*

	Nursing Diagnoses	**Collaborative Problems and Medical Diagnoses**
Focus of Assessment Activities	Main focus is upon monitoring human responses to actual and potential health problems.	Main focus is on monitoring for *pathophysiologic response* of body organs or systems.
Problem Identification	Nurse identifies and validates that problem exists independently.	Nurse may identify problem but is required to refer to physician for validation that problem exists (may require additional diagnostic studies to label the problem). Nurse may not be qualified to diagnose exact nature of problem, but refers abnormal data to the physician.
Treatment	Nurse initiates interventions for treatment independently.	Nurse collaborates with physician to initiate interventions for treatment. Nurse may have standing orders from physician or institution (delegated authority) to initiate diagnostic studies or treatment interventions for the problem without physician's orders.

☐ *Practice Session*   *Nursing Diagnoses and Collaborative Problems*
(Suggested Answers on page 171)

For the following problems, write ND in front of those that are nursing diagnoses and CP in front of those that are collaborative problems. (For each problem, ask yourself, "Can the nurse independently initiate the major interventions for this problem?" If the answer is "yes," label it ND. If the answer is "no," label it CP.)

1. _CP_ Potential complication: hemorrhage secondary to clotting problems
2. _ND_ Potential Ineffective Airway Clearance related to copious secretions
3. _ND_ Potential for Injury related to generalized weakness
4. _CP_ Potential complication: fluid volume overload secondary to intravenous therapy.
5. _CP_ Fluid Volume Deficit related to insufficient fluid intake
6. _ND_ Impaired Skin Integrity related to pressure points
7. _CP_ Potential complication: cardiac arrhythmias secondary to potassium deficiency
8. _CP_ Potential complication: septicemia secondary to central venous line
9. _ND_ Diversional Activity Deficit related to prescribed bedrest
10. _CP_ Potential complication: increased intracranial pressure secondary to concussion
11. _ND_ Potential complication: malnutrition secondary to prescribed NPO
12. _ND_ Altered Nutrition: Less than Body Requirements related to poor appetite
13. _ND_ Impaired Physical Mobility related to prescribed bedrest
14. _CP_ Potential complication: pneumothorax secondary to chest tube
15. _CP_ Potential complication: thrombus formation secondary to venous shunt placement.

Working With the NANDA List of Nursing Diagnoses

Most nurses have found the accepted list of nursing diagnoses published by NANDA to be very helpful in identifying nursing diagnoses. However, some have been frustrated with "having to learn new terms for old problems." Others find some of the new terms difficult to understand and wonder where they fit into their clinical practice. Perhaps all this is because many nurses have been confused about the purpose of the NANDA list.

NANDA has been clear that when it publishes its accepted list every two years, it is publishing *diagnostic labels that have been accepted for clinical testing*. This means that some initial studies have been done for each diagnostic label, but each requires further clinical testing and research to validate that it is indeed a problem that can be identified and treated by nurses. The NANDA list is a beginning list of *suggested terms* for *suggested health problems* that may be identified and treated by nurses.

Each of the diagnostic category labels accepted by NANDA consists of three components: title, defining characteristics, and etiological or related factors. These components are described:

☐ **Title (or label):** Offers a concise description of the health problem

☐ **Defining characteristics:** Cluster of signs and symptoms that are often seen with that particular diagnosis

☐ **Etiological and contributing factors:** Identifies those situational, pathophysiological, and maturational factors that can cause or contribute to the problem

For examples of a category label with corresponding etiologies and defining characteristics, check the Nursing Diagnosis Quick Reference Section in the back of this book. You will find that some of the diagnoses are well defined, while others need more work. There are "holes" in the list, especially in specialty areas. However, we *do* have a beginning, and most nurses are finding many of the diagnostic labels to be helpful in labeling the problems that they identify and treat independently. Those of you who become frustrated with changes in terminology and additions to the list should remember the following:

☐ You do not have to use every diagnosis on the list. Use those that apply to your practice.

☐ If the problem you've identified is not on the list, you can write your own nursing diagnoses using the Guidelines on page 78.

☐ Change is a part of evolution and, ultimately, *progress.* (Nursing, unlike medicine, is just beginning to develop its terminology for diagnoses. What would have happened to medicine if physicians had said "Oh, no! Now they're telling us that *cancer* can have many different names . . . Why can't they just stick with *cancer*?" Or better yet: "Oh, no! Now they've added this new diagnosis, *AIDS*, to the list . . . don't we have enough diagnoses already?")

While we can expect changes (additions, deletions, and modification of category label names), we must realize the importance of the work of NANDA and the need to continue to work together to develop a common terminology. Although it will take time to validate which diagnoses are useful, and which diagnoses need to be deleted or refined, the current list is an important *starting point* for the use of nursing diagnoses for the following reasons:

☐ Using a nationally accepted list of diagnoses will help nurses to communicate with each other using common terminology. Nursing knowledge will be easier to learn and teach if authors, faculty, and clinicians all use the same terminology. (Imagine if physicians could use any word they wanted to describe pneumonia!)

☐ Using common terminology will facilitate the use of computers for nursing. (Nurses will be able to retrieve records according to nursing diagnoses rather than medical diagnoses, and therefore will be able to collect data to further research in nursing.)

☐ Using a nationally accepted list of diagnostic categories provides a method for reimbursement according to nursing activities related to nursing diagnoses rather than just medical diagnoses. (Two people with the same medical diagnosis do not necessarily have the same *nursing* needs.)

☐ All nurses can work together toward testing and refining the diagnostic categories to identify assessment criteria and nursing interventions that nurses can use to improve nursing care.

> **Note:** This chapter focuses on identifying nursing diagnoses both by using the NANDA-accepted list and by generating your own specific nursing diagnoses. It is this author's philosophy that *if you can use NANDA terminology to define the nursing diagnosis, you should use their terms.* If you cannot find a diagnosis on the list that accurately describes the health problem that you have identified, then write your own nursing diagnosis using the guidelines set forth in this chapter.

Writing Diagnostic Statements for Actual Nursing Diagnoses

Now that we have examined the NANDA list and how it affects nursing at a national level, let's take a look at how to write diagnostic statements for the nursing diagnoses that you identify in your practice.

When you write a diagnostic statement for an actual nursing diagnosis, you should use the PES (problem, etiology, signs and symptoms) system to describe the diagnosis. That is, you write a three-part statement which includes the following:

1. The problem (P)
2. Its cause or etiology (E)
3. The signs and symptoms (defining characteristics) that are evident in the patient (S)

The PES format applies the basic principle of stating the problem and its etiology, and adds the concept of validation. When you read such a diagnostic statement, you know *the problem, its etiology, and the signs and symptoms* that lead the diagnostician to believe that the problem exists.

Including signs and symptoms in the diagnostic statement *validates* why you chose a specific diagnosis. For example, if you read that a patient has *Ineffective Airway Clearance related to incisional pain,* you do not know for sure what made the nurse choose that diagnostic label. However, if you read *Ineffective Airway Clearance related to incisional pain as manifested by poor cough effort and statements that incision hurts too much to cough,* you have a clear picture of why the nurse chose that particular diagnosis.

To write a statement which validates an actual nursing diagnosis, remember the following rule:

> **Rule:** *To write a diagnostic statement for an actual nursing diagnosis,* link the problem and its etiology by using "related to." Add "as manifested by" or "as evidenced by," and state the major signs and symptoms that validate that the diagnosis exists. *Example: Impaired Communication related to inability to speak English as manifested by inability to follow instructions in English and verbalization of requests in Spanish.*

Display 3-8 summarizes the components of a three-part statement for actual nursing diagnoses.

Display 3-8. Three-Part Diagnostic Statement for Actual Nursing Diagnoses

1. Health problem: Ineffective Airway Clearance
                                                                          ↓
                                                                   related to

2. Etiology: weak cough and incisional pain
                                                                          ↓
                                                              as manifested by

3. Signs and symptoms   poor or no cough effort and statements that
   (defining characteristics):   incision hurts too much when he coughs

Diagnostic statement: *Ineffective Airway Clearance related to weak cough and incisional pain,* as manifested by poor or no cough effort and statements that incision hurts too much when he coughs

---

☐ *Practice Session*   *Using the PES Format to Validate Actual Nursing Diagnoses*
                        (Suggested Answers on page 171)

Read all of the data for each of the case histories below and write a three-part diagnostic statement that clearly describes the diagnosis.

1. Mr. Starr has the following signs and symptoms:

Chronic cough productive of mucus

States he has smoked three packs of cigarettes a day for 15 years

Smokes constantly in his room

Elevated arterial CO_2

You identify the diagnosis of *Impaired Gas Exchange.*

2. Bob O'Brien has the following signs and symptoms:

States he has had no appetite for 2 weeks

You have recorded a 10-lb weight loss.

He weighs 15 lb less than his recommended weight.

You identify the diagnosis of *Altered Nutrition: Less Than Body Requirements.*

3. Lilly Johns has the following signs and symptoms:

She is unable to move either leg.

She has limited passive range of motion in lower joints.

You identify the diagnosis of *Impaired Physical Mobility.*

Writing Diagnostic Statements for Potential and Possible Nursing Diagnoses

If you assess your patient and note that there are some high-risk factors present that may cause him to have a certain nursing diagnosis, then you have identified a potential nursing diagnosis. For example, suppose you were taking care of an elderly woman who was very thin, immobile, and bedridden. She may have had excellent care at home, and as a result has beautiful, healthy looking skin. However, you should be aware that her age, weight, immobility, and confinement to bed can be contributing or etiological factors for *Impaired Skin Integrity*. You should then document the potential nursing diagnosis by writing a two-part statement that describes both the problem and its cause (*e.g.*, *Potential Impaired Skin Integrity* related to advanced age, immobility, and confinement to bed). You would then establish a plan of care that would prevent irritated or broken skin (*e.g.*, establish a regimen of monitoring for pressure points and of turning, repositioning, and massaging to promote circulation to the skin). Remember the following rule:

> **Rule:** *To write a diagnostic statement for a potential nursing diagnosis*, write a two-part statement by stating the potential problem and adding "related to" to link the problem and the contributing factors (risk factors). *Example: Potential for Injury related to blindness.**

If you suspect a nursing diagnosis, but do not have enough information to be sure, you should label it as a *possible nursing diagnosis*. If you suspect a specific cause for the problem, you should write a two-part statement by stating the possible diagnosis and the contributing factors (*e.g.*, *Possible Spiritual Distress related to terminal cancer*). Your plan of care would then include interventions *to gather more information* to determine whether the diagnosis is actually present. Remember the following rule.

> **Rule:** *To write a diagnostic statement for a possible diagnosis*, write a two-part statement by stating the possible problem and adding "related to" to link it with the possible contributing factors. *Example: Possible Sexual Patterns related to partner's diagnosis of Herpes.*

Display 3-9 on page 75 summarizes how to write two-part and three-part diagnostic statements. Table 3-2 below it compares actual, potential, and possible nursing diagnoses.

☐ *Practice Session*   *Writing Diagnostic Statements for Potential and Possible Nursing Diagnoses*
(*Suggested Answers on page 171*)

Read the data for each of the case histories below and write a two-part diagnostic statement that clearly describes the diagnosis.

1. Mr. Reardon has been confined to bed with casts on both his legs. He seems

* You do not write "as manifested by" for a potential diagnosis because if there were evidence that the diagnosis existed (*i.e.*, signs and symptoms), you would have an *actual* nursing diagnosis.

angry and has stated that he does not want to talk to anyone. You are aware that he has had a fight with his girlfriend. You suspect that he may have the diagnosis of *Ineffective Individual Coping related to confinement to bed or possibly problems with significant others.* However, you are not sure if Mr. Reardon's withdrawal is a temporary method of coping that works for him.

NURSING DIAGNOSIS:

2. Mr. Cappelli has a temperature of 101°F. He sleeps a lot and has a poor appetite. He drinks about 2000 ml a day if you offer frequent fluids and encourage him to drink. You recognize that fever is a contributing factor for *Fluid Volume Deficit.*

NURSING DIAGNOSIS:

3. Mr. Rogers has just had his gallbladder removed today under general anesthesia. His nursing assessment form has documented that he has smoked a pack of cigarettes a day for the past 20 years. He has no productive cough at present, but you recognize that his smoking and recent general anesthesia are contributing factors for *Ineffective Airway Clearance.*

NURSING DIAGNOSIS:

4. You see Mrs. Jackson in clinic 6 weeks after a hysterectomy. She states that she feels well physically, but that emotionally, she just does not feel like herself yet. She states that she gets angry easily and cries a lot. She states that she feels that she gets no support from her husband. You note that her nursing assessment form from her admission to the hospital for the hysterectomy 6 weeks ago recorded that she had expressed concern about the effect of hysterectomies on sexual functions. You suspect that she may have the diagnosis of *Sexual Dysfunction.*

NURSING DIAGNOSIS:

> ### Display 3-9.   Writing Two-Part and Three-Part Diagnostic Statements
>
> 1. Actual nursing diagnosis (three-part statement):
>
> | Problem + Etiology + Signs and symptoms present |
> | --- |
>
> EXAMPLE:
>
> *Self-care Deficit related to inability to move both arms as manifested by casts on both hands and wrists*
>
> 2. Potential and possible nursing diagnoses (two-part statement):
>
> | Problem + Etiology |
> | --- |
>
> EXAMPLES:
>
> *Potential Ineffective Airway Clearance related to smoking*
>
> *Possible Disturbance in Self-concept related to chronic illness*

Table 3-2.   Comparison of Actual, Potential, and Possible Nursing Diagnoses

Nursing Diagnosis	Signs and Symptoms Present?	Etiological/ Contributing Factors Present?	Nursing Plan
Actual nursing diagnosis	Yes	Yes	Monitor signs and symptoms present to determine improvements or deterioration in condition. Identify interventions to reduce or eliminate the cause of the problem.
Potential nursing diagnosis	No	Yes	Perform daily focus assessments to determine if signs and symptoms have appeared to change status from *potential* to *actual*. Identify interventions to prevent, reduce, or remove contributing factors.
Possible nursing diagnosis	Unsure	Unsure	Gather more data to clarify vague cues and to determine if the signs and symptoms or contributing factors are actually present.

(Adapted with permission from Carpenito L: Unpublished workshop notes, 1985)

Focusing Analysis to Identify Nursing Diagnoses

In the first part of this chapter, basic principles and steps for diagnostic reasoning were presented. Now we will apply these principles and steps to help you focus your analysis to identify nursing diagnoses.

Identifying Usual Lifestyles and Coping Patterns

An important aspect of identifying nursing diagnoses is that of identifying usual lifestyles and coping patterns. This is because nursing diagnoses focus upon *how the individual is affected* by health problems, and how the individual can attain or maintain an optimal health state *in his own way.* If you understand the person's lifestyle (what he does most days, what he likes to do, what he does not like to do, and how he views his health state), you will be better able to understand how a given health problem is affecting the individual's sense of well-being. Learning about a person's lifestyle may also help to identify some factors that are actually contributing to the problem. For example, you may find out that a person who has chronic constipation hates to exercise and lives an exceedingly sedentary life, which could contribute to the constipation.

Identifying how a person usually copes with changes in lifestyle helps to determine how the person might be able to deal with the health problem. For example, a person who likes to do physical exercise or work when he is depressed may find confinement to a bed more difficult than a person who simply likes to read to get his mind off his problems.

The following are some questions to ask that may help you in identifying how an individual's daily life may be affected by a given health problem, and whether the person will be able to cope with necessary changes to optimize his health state.

☐ How do you think this problem has changed (will change) you daily life?

☐ How do you feel you have coped (will cope) with these changes?

☐ Tell me how you usually adapt to change.

☐ What is the worst thing about having this problem (making these changes)?

☐ Do you have resources (personal, community) that have helped (can help) you cope better?

Determining the Etiology of Nursing Diagnoses

As stated earlier, it is as important to learn how to identify the etiology of a problem as it is to identify the problem itself.

Just as with problem identification, identifying etiologies depends on the individual nurse's nursing knowledge, experience, and analytical skills. Learning to identify etiologies will become easier as you grow in theoretical and practical nursing knowledge. However, there are some questions that you can ask to help in identifying etiologies. Consider the questions listed below.

☐ What are the factors that the client (or family) identifies as causing or contributing to the problem?

☐ Are there factors related to developmental age, presence of disease, or situational changes in lifestyle that could be contributing to the problem?

☐ Have your other resources for data collection and analysis (medical records, other healthcare professionals, literature review) identified some factors that might be causing or contributing to the problem?

Identifying Nursing Diagnoses On the NANDA List

The NANDA list of nursing diagnoses provides assistance to nurses who are learning to label nursing diagnoses. Let's take a look at how to use the list to help you identify nursing diagnoses.

☐ *Guidelines*   *Learning How to Identify NANDA-Accepted Nursing Diagnoses*

☐ Become familiar with the list.

1. Study the list and choose some diagnoses that you believe you will encounter frequently, and learn these first. For example, *Constipation, Potential Impaired Skin Integrity, Fear,* and *Anxiety* are diagnoses that even beginning nursing students are able to identify.

2. Do not feel that you have to use every diagnosis on the list. If you are philosophically opposed to using a certain diagnosis, throw that diagnosis out, but not the entire list.

3. Organize the list so that related diagnoses are listed together, *e.g.,* problems with respiration, problems with elimination, *etc.* (See the inside front cover for NANDA organization (Unitary Person), its facing page for organization of diagnoses according to Functional Health Patterns, and the Nursing Diagnosis Quick Reference Section for an alphabetical list of nursing diagnoses.)

☐ Follow the steps for identifying nursing diagnoses/problems.

1. Practice using focus assessment tools that help to gather specific data for each particular diagnosis.*

2. Gather, interpret, and cluster your signs and symptoms (objective and subjective data).

---

* Specific focus assessment criteria questions for each nursing diagnosis category can be found in Carpenito, L. (1989) *Nursing Diagnosis: Application to Clinical Practice.* 3rd Ed. Philadelphia: JB Lippincott.

3. Be aware of medical diagnoses present because certain nursing diagnoses are frequently associated with certain medical diagnoses (*e.g.*, people with diabetes have a high potential for Impaired Skin Integrity).

4. Study the signs and symptoms that you have clustered together, and choose a diagnostic label that seems to describe the problem. *Compare the signs and symptoms with the defining characteristics for that particular diagnostic category.* All of the defining characteristics need not be present, but at least one should be evident in order to confirm the diagnosis.

5. Be specific when you use an accepted diagnostic label. Use qualifying or quantifying adjectives when appropriate. (*e.g.*, mild, moderate, severe).

6. If the diagnostic category is followed by the word "specify" use a colon and specify the area where the problem occurs. For example, if you identify *Knowledge Deficit*, you must specify in what area the person needs to learn (*e.g.*, *Knowledge Deficit: Side Effects of Medications*).

Identifying Nursing Diagnoses That Are Not On the NANDA List

The NANDA list of nursing diagnoses is incomplete. Therefore, you may find that you identify a problem that you feel should be considered to be a nursing diagnosis, and yet you may not be able to find a category label on the list that describes it appropriately. The following guidelines are suggested for labeling a nursing diagnosis that is not on the suggested list.

☐ *Guidelines*   *Identifying Nursing Diagnoses Not On the NANDA List*

1. Gather, interpret, and cluster your signs and symptoms (objective and subjective data).

2. Be sure that you are not renaming a medical diagnosis or problem. If it is a medical problem, or collaborative problem, say so. (For example, call hypotension by its own name. Do not rename it "alteration in hemodynamics.")

3. Be sure that you have not made any of the common errors for stating nursing diagnoses. (See Guidelines: Avoiding Errors When Writing Diagnostic Statements.)

4. Be sure that none of the NANDA category labels are appropriate to describe the problem.

5. State the problem and its etiology and list the defining characteristics for this particular patient using the PES format, if possible.

EXAMPLE:

Destructive Behavior related to poor role model at home as manifested by playing with matches and abusing school property

Using Nursing Diagnosis Terminology Correctly

Learning how to write diagnostic statements that clearly define both the problem and its etiology can be difficult at first. The following guidelines are suggested to help prevent errors.

☐ *Guidelines*   *Avoiding Errors When Writing Diagnostic Statements*

☐ Don't state the nursing diagnosis in medical terminology.

EXAMPLE:

Incorrect: Mastectomy related to cancer
Correct: Potential Altered Self-concept related to mastectomy

☐ Don't state the nursing diagnosis as a medical diagnosis.

EXAMPLE:

Incorrect: Potential for pneumonia
Correct: Ineffective Airway Clearance related to poor cough effort.

☐ Don't state two problems at the same time.

EXAMPLE:

Incorrect: Pain and Fear related to diagnostic procedures
Correct: Fear related to unfamiliarity with diagnostic procedures
        Pain related to diagnostic procedures

☐ Don't write the diagnostic statement in such a way that it may be legally incriminating.

EXAMPLE:

Incorrect: Potential for Injury related to lack of siderails on bed
Correct: Potential for Injury related to disorientation

☐ Don't "rename" a medical problem to make it a nursing diagnosis

EXAMPLE:

Incorrect: Alteration in Hemodynamics related to hypovolemia
Correct: Hypovolemia. (This is a medical problem, rather than a nursing diagnosis, and you should use medical terminology to describe this problem.)

☐ Don't write a nursing diagnosis based on value judgments.

EXAMPLE:

Incorrect: Spiritual Distress related to atheism as manifested by statements that he has never believed in God
Correct: There may be no diagnosis in this situation. The person may be at peace with his beliefs (not with yours).

☐ *Practice Session*   *Identifying Correctly Stated Nursing Diagnoses*
(Suggested Answers to page 171)

For each of the nursing diagnostic statements listed below, put C in front of the ones that are correctly stated.

1. __C__ Potential Constipation related to bedrest
2. _____ Potential Malnutrition
3. _____ Potential Pneumonia
4. __e__ Need for increased fluids related to thirst
5. __C__ Ineffective Individual Coping related to sensory bombardment
6. __C__ Potential Fluid Volume Deficit related to fever and sore throat
7. _____ Lung cancer related to metastasis
8. __C__ Altered Self-concept related to mastectomy
9. __C__ Anxiety related to unknown etiology
10. _____ Infection related to burns
11. _____ Altered Communication
12. _____ Sudden Infant Death Syndrome related to low birth weight
13. __C__ Potential Violence related to inability to vent anger
14. _____ Altered Urinary Elimination related to Foley catheter
15. __C__ Altered Urinary Elimination related to bedwetting

Diagnostic Statements for Collaborative Problems

Collaborative problems are not written on the nursing care plan unless the situation is unusual. This is because the nursing interventions for collaborative problems are usually determined by hospital policies, procedures, and standards, or by physicians' orders. For example, suppose you have a patient with an intravenous (IV) line. This would be considered a collaborative problem because it is necessary to have a physician's order for initiation of treatment,

---

* The *"as evidenced by"* or *"as manifested by"* to validate these diagnoses has been omitted.

and usually hospital policies will direct care and assessment of IV lines. Writing these types of problems on the care plan would be redundant and time consuming; you would be less likely to focus on the unique nursing problems if you took the time to list all of the collaborative problems. For these reasons, a collaborative problem should not be written on the nursing care plan unless the problem is unusual, or if it's not addressed by hospital policies or physicians' orders.

While you will not be writing most collaborative problems on the care plan, you may be asked to describe a collaborative problem. Carpenito (1987) stresses the importance of having *common terminology to describe collaborative problems*. She suggests using the term *potential complication*. For example, if your patient has an IV, you might describe the following:

> *Potential complications: thrombus/phlebitis/infiltration/fluid overload, secondary to IV*

Using the term *potential complication* focuses the problem statement on *the complication that may occur* because of the disease, trauma, or diagnostic or treatment situation. This type of focusing will help you to determine what complications you are looking for, and may also suggest how the complications might be prevented. For example, note how statement *a* below will better direct you in determining nursing assessment and interventions than statement *b*.

> a. Potential complication: arrhythmias secondary to low serum potassium
> b. Collaborative problem: arrhythmias

Statement *a* tells you that you will have to monitor for (and prevent) low serum potassium. Statement *a* also applies basic principles of diagnostic reasoning and *states both the problem and its cause*. Remember the following rule:

Rule: Whenever possible, describe collaborative problems using the term *potential complication*. Link the problem and its cause by using "secondary to" or "related to." *Example: Potential Complication: Paralytic ileus secondary to back surgery.*

Table 3-3 lists examples of collaborative problems that nurses frequently encounter in the medical–surgical area.

Identifying Collaborative Problems (Potential Complications)

Your ability to identify collaborative problems (potential complications) will depend on your knowledge of disease process, trauma, surgery, anesthesia, and diagnostic and treatment modalities. If you don't have knowledge of

Table 3-3. *Common Collaborative Problems*

Source of Problem	Collaborative Problem

Intravenous therapy	Potential complications:
	  Phlebitis
	  IV infiltration
	  Fluid overload

Nasogastric suction	Potential complications:
	  Occlusion of nasogastric tube
	  Electrolyte imbalance

Skeletal traction/casts	Potential complication:
	  Poor alignment of bones
	  Bleeding
	  Swelling
	  Compromised circulation
	  Neuropathology

Medications	Potential complications:
	  Side-effects
	  Adverse reaction/allergy
	  Overdosage

Foley catheter	Potential complications: Blockage of the catheter

Chest tubes	Potential complications:
	  Blockage of the chest tube
	  Hemo/pneumothorax
	  Bleeding
	  Atelectasis

Surgery/trauma	Potential complications:
	  Atelectasis
	  Bleeding/shock/hypovolemia
	  Electrolyte imbalance
	  Paralytic ileus
	  Oliguria/anuria
	  Shock/hypovolemia
	  Fluid overload/congestive heart
	    failure

Head trauma	Potential complications:
	  Bleeding/shock
	  Brain swelling
	  Increased intracranial pressure
	  Coma

potential complications, you should have readily available a reference (*e.g.*, medical–surgical text, obstetric text) that will provide this information for you. By keeping this reference available, and by consulting with more qualified professionals, you will be better able to identify potential complications.

The following guidelines will help you identify potential complications (collaborative problems).

☐ *Guidelines*   *Identifying Potential Complications (Collaborative Problems)*

1. Consider your patient's medical diagnosis and determine the signs and symptoms of the *most frequent and most dangerous complications*.
2. Be aware of recent diagnostic or treatment modalities, and determine whether there are associated potential complications.
3. If the situation is complex, check with a reference or a more qualified professional (*e.g.*, ask the attending physician or a clinical nurse specialist, "There is a lot going on with this patient. Are there any *specific complications* that we should be looking for?")
4. Consult policy, procedures, protocols, and standards that address your patient's diagnostic or treatment situations (*e.g.*, management of chest tubes), because they will often list associated potential complications.

☐ *Practice Session*   *Identifying Strengths, Nursing Diagnoses, and Collaborative Problems* (*Suggested Answers on page 171*)

Study the data given for each of the following case histories. On a separate piece of paper list the strengths, nursing diagnoses, and collaborative problems that you can identify (actual, potential, possible). Use the PES format to validate your diagnoses.

Case History A (Mrs. Goode, 31 years old)

Medical Diagnosis: Cerebral concussion

Subjective Data

  States she was hit on the head by a falling branch

  States she has a headache and feels dizzy when she lifts her head off the pillow

  Expressed concern about having her husband look after her two children because "he is not good with them"

  States she is afraid of hospitals and needles

States she has never worked outside the home because her children need her

States "I can't stay in bed and use the bedpan as the doctor said"

Objective Data

Age: 31; Ht: 5'3"; Wt: 160 lb

Nursing Physical Assessment

Temperature: 98.4°F

Pulse: 78 and regular

Respirations: 24 and nonlabored

Blood Pressure: 128/72

Moves all extremities with equal strength

Pupils are equally reactive to light

Large bruise over right forehead

Abdomen soft, nontender, obese

Peripheral pulses strong

IV in right arm looks red and infiltrated.

Case History B (Mr. Northe, 54 years old)

Medical Diagnosis: Atrial fibrillation/rule out myocardial infarction

Subjective Data

States this is his second "heart attack", and is well aware of rationale afor medications

States that he is "worried about being in bed for 3 weeks like last time"

Complains of mild chest discomfort in the substernal area, says "it feels like gas"

Says he is glad he has good insurance for his wife and family—his brother, who was only 2 years older, died of a heart attack last year

Complains of having had no appetite for 3 days, and that he hasn't had a bowel movement in 5 days

States he hates being on bedrest because he gets "stiff all over from not moving"

Objective Data

Age: 54; Ht: 5'11"; Wt: 160 lb

Nursing Physical Assessment

Temperature: 97.8°F

Pulse: 64 and irregular (monitor shows atrial fibrillation without PVCs)

Respirations: 32

Blood Pressure: 140/92

Skin: warm, dry, and pink

Lungs: a few scattered rales at bases

Oxygen on at 4 liters/min via cannula

Becomes easily short of breath

Peripheral pulses satisfactory/Circulation with good capillary refill

IV with potassium in left arm at 100 ml/hr

Intake last 24 hours = 2400 ml

Output last 24 hours = 1000 ml

Note two red pressure areas on both heels

Figure 3-1 illustrates the diagnostic process, beginning with assessment and culminating with identification of client strengths, nursing diagnoses, and collaborative problems.

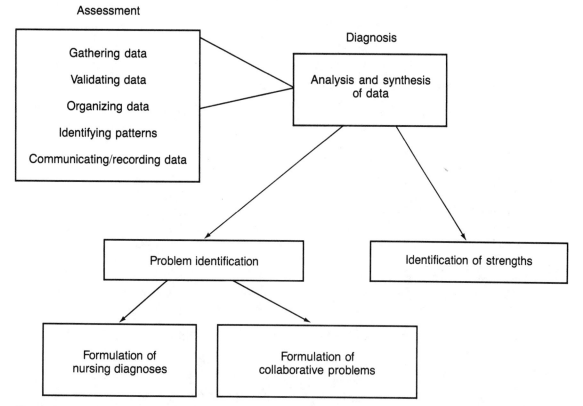

Figure 3-1. *The diagnostic process.*

1. Although there are varying views on defining nursing diagnosis, on whether to include healthy responses as diagnoses, and on whether pathophysiologic responses should be labeled nursing diagnoses, there is a consensus that *nurses do indeed diagnose health problems.*

2. Diagnosis involves putting key pieces of data together to identify actual and potential health problems (which will be the basis of the plan of care) and strengths (which will be utilized and reinforced when developing the plan of care).

3. Your ability to apply principles and steps of diagnostic reasoning will assist you to identify health problems with a greater degree of safety and accuracy.

4. *Diagnostic reasoning* can include the use of *intuition* to expedite problem identification, as long as you know how to act safely upon feelings of "knowing something without evidence."

5. Nursing diagnoses differ from collaborative problems in both focus and responsibility:

   □ Nursing diagnoses focus more on the *human responses* than the disease, and nurses are responsible for identifying and treating them *independently.*

   □ Collaborative problems focus more on *the pathophysiologic response of organs or systems,* and nurses are responsible for identifying and treating them *in collaboration with the physician.*

6. Medical diagnoses are collaborative problems *for the nurse* (*i.e.,* the nurse focuses on detecting potential complications of the diagnoses).

7. *Collaborative problems* are not written on the care plan unless they are unusual or complex, because nursing interventions for their care are usually addressed by hospital policies, procedures, standards, or physicians' orders.

8. The NANDA list is a beginning list of *suggested terms for suggested health problems* that may be identified and treated by nurses. (NANDA requests nurses to research and test the diagnoses that seem useful, and to submit results to NANDA for consideration.)

9. Each of the diagnoses listed by NANDA has three components:

   □ The category label (problem)

   □ The defining characteristics (cluster of signs, symptoms, and risk factors often seen with the diagnosis)

   □ The common etiologies for the problem

10. You should use NANDA terminology to describe the diagnoses that you have identified whenever possible. However, if you diagnose a health problem that can be treated independently, but cannot find a category label on the NANDA list that adequately describes this problem, you should write the nursing diagnosis in your own terms, using the PES format.

11. When writing a diagnostic statement for *actual* nursing diagnoses, you should write a three-part statement using the PES format.

    EXAMPLE:

    Impaired Verbal Communication related to inability to speak English as manifested by inability to follow instructions in English and verbalizing requests in Spanish

12. When writing a diagnostic statement for a *potential* or *possible* nursing diagnosis, you should write a two-part statement that describes both the problem and its etiology, when known.

    EXAMPLES:

    Potential for Fear related to bad previous experience of being left alone at night

    Possible Knowledge Deficit: Colostomy care

13. When writing a problem statement for a collaborative problem you should use the word "potential complication" to clearly describe the collaborative problem. If adding "related to" or "secondary to" clarifies the problem, then also add the etiology.

    EXAMPLES:

    Potential complication: Heart block related to digitalis toxicity

    Potential complication: Fat emboli secondary to fractured femur

Bibliography

American Nurses' Association (1980) *Nursing: A Social Policy Statement.* Kansas City, MO.

American Nurses' Association (1973) *Standards of Nursing Practice.* Kansas City. MO.

Berger, M. (1984) Clinical thinking ability and nursing students. *Journal of Nursing Education* 23(7):306–308.

Berry, K. (1987) Let's create diagnoses psych nurses can use. *Am. J. Nurs.* 87:797–798.

Carnevali, D. (1983) *Nursing Care Planning: Diagnosis and Management.* Philadelphia: JB Lippincott.

Carnevali, D., Mitchell, P., Woods, N., and Tanner, C. (1984) *Diagnostic Reasoning in Nursing.* Philadelphia: JB Lippincott.

Carpenito, L. (1987) *Nursing Diagnosis: Application to Clinical Practice.* 2nd ed. Philadelphia: JB Lippincott.

Carpenito, L. (1987) *Handbook of Nursing Diagnosis.* 2nd ed. Philadelphia: JB Lippincott.

Carpenito, L. (1984) Is the problem a nursing diagnosis? *Am. J. Nurs.* 84(11):1418–1419.

Carpenito, L. (1985) Diagnosing nutrition problems. *Am. J. Nurs.* 85(5):584.

Carpenito, L. (1985) Diagnostics: Actual, potential, or possible nursing diagnoses. *Am. J. Nurs.* 85(4):458.

Carpenito, L. (1985) Nursing diagnosis: Selected dilemmas in practice. *Occupational Health Nursing.* August:397–400.

Creason, N. (1987) How do we define nursing diagnosis? *Am. J. Nurs.* 87:230–231.

Gordon, M. (1985) Nursing diagnosis annual review. *Nursing Research* 3:127–146.

Gordon, M. (1987) *Nursing Diagnosis: Process and Application.* New York: McGraw–Hill Co.

Guzzetta, C. and Kinney, M. (1986) Mastering the transition from medical to nursing diagnosis. *Progress in Cardiovascular Nursing* 1:43–44.

Guzzetta, K., Bunton, S., Prinkey, L., Sherer, A., and Seifert, P. (1988) Unitary person assessment tool: Easing the problems with nursing diagnoses. *Focus* 15(2):12–24.

Houldin, A. (1987) *Nursing Diagnoses for Wellness: Supporting Strengths.* Philadelphia: JB Lippincott.

Hurley, M. (ed). (1986) *Classification of Nursing Diagnoses: Proceedings of the Sixth Conference.* St. Louis: CV Mosby.

Kim, M. and Moritz, D. (1987) Classification of Nursing Diagnoses/Proceedings of the Third and Fourth National Conference. New York: McGraw–Hill Co.

Kim, M. McFarland, G., and McLane, A. (1984) *Classification of Nursing Diagnoses: Proceedings of the Fifth Conference.* St. Louis: CV Mosby.

Kriteck, P. (1985) Nursing diagnosis in perspective: Response to a critique. *Image* 17:3–8.

LaFortune, F. (1988) Common diagnostic errors. *Nurs Educator* 13(3):31–35.

McFarland, G. and Wasli, L. (1986) *Nursing Diagnoses and Process in Mental Health Nursing.* Philadelphia: JB Lippincott.

Moritz, D. (1984) Nursing diagnosis in relation to the nursing process. In Kim, M. and Moritz, D. (eds.): *Classification of Nursing Diagnoses/Proceedings of the Third and Fourth National Conferences.* New York: McGraw–Hill.

North American Nursing Diagnosis Association (1987) *Taxonomy I.* St. Louis, MO.

Nursing diagnosis (1984) *Top. Clin. Nurs.* 5:1–96.

Nursing diagnosis (1984) *AORN J* 40(8).

Nursing diagnosis (1985) *Nurs. Clin. North. Am.* 20(4).

Nursing diagnosis (1985) *Occup. Health. Nurs.* 33.

Polit, D. and Hungler, B. (1987) *Nursing Research: Principles and Methods.* 3rd ed. Philadelphia: JB Lippincott.

Soares, C. (1978) Nursing and medical diagnoses: A comparison of variant and essential features. In Chaska, N. (ed): *The Nursing Profession: Views Through the Mist.* New York: McGraw–Hill.

Stolte, K. (1986) A complementary view of nursing diagnosis. *Public Health Nursing* 3(1):23–28.

Stolte, K. (1986) Nursing diagnoses and the childbearing woman. *Maternal Child Nursing* 11(1):13–15.

Wake, M. (ed). (1987) Symposium: Nursing diagnosis in critical care. *Heart and Lung* 16(6):593–635.

Vaughan–Wroble, B. and Perkins, S. (1986) Nursing diagnosis: The pivotal point of the nursing process in cardiovascular nursing. *Cardiovascular Nursing* 5(22):25–29.

Ziegler, S., Vaughan–Wroble, B., and Erlen, J. (1986) *Nursing Process, Nursing Diagnosis, Nursing Knowledge: Avenues to Autonomy.* Norwalk, CT: Appleton–Lange.

☑ Setting Priorities
☑ Establishing Goals
☑ Determining Nursing Interventions
☑ Documenting the Plan of Care

4
Planning

Standard III: *The plan of nursing care includes goals derived from the nursing diagnoses.*

Standard IV: *The plan of nursing care includes priorities and the prescribed nursing approaches or measures to achieve the goals derived from nursing diagnoses.*

Standard V: *Nursing actions provide for client/patient participation in health promotion, maintenance, and restoration.*

Standard VI: *Nursing actions assist the client/patient to maximize his health capabilities.**

*Abstracted from Standards of Nursing Practice. Copyright American Nurses' Association, 1973

Client-Centered Goal (or Outcome) A client (or patient) objective that describes measurable data that tell you whether the individual has achieved the expected benefit of nursing care. For example, *"The client will demonstrate effective airway clearance as evidenced by clear lungs, ability to bring forth sputum with cough, and absence of fever."*

Long-Term Goal An objective that is expected to be achieved over a relatively long period of time, usually weeks or months.

Measurable Verb Verbs that describe an exact behavior that you can *see* or *hear*.

Nursing Care Plan A written plan of nursing care that describes nursing diagnoses, expected outcomes, nursing orders, and client progress.

Nursing Order A statement written by the nurse that specifies nursing interventions that all nurses caring for that specific patient should follow.

Nursing Standard A statement or protocol that describes how a nurse should give nursing care in a certain situation (determined by laws, the ANA, and by each individual healthcare facility).

POMR (Problem-Oriented Medical Records) A method of documenting a patient's care whereby all healthcare professionals caring for a given patient chart the identified problems in the same place, using SOAP forms.

Short-Term Goal A goal that is expected to be achieved in a relatively short period of time, usually less than a week.

SOAP Charting A method of documenting a plan of care by charting the following data:

S = Subjective data
O = Objective data
A = Assessment (problem statement)
P = Plan (goals)

SOAPIE Charting A method of documenting a plan of care by charting the following data:

S = Subjective data
O = Objective data
A = Assessment (problem statement)
P = Plan (goals)
I = Interventions
E = Evaluation

Planning: Determining Priorities, Goals, and Interventions

Once you have identified specific nursing diagnoses and collaborative problems you are ready to begin the third step of the nursing process: *planning*. This is the time when you will determine how to give nursing care in an organized, individualized, goal-directed manner. Planning will involve the following:

☐ Setting priorities

☐ Establishing client goals/expected outcomes

☐ Determining nursing actions/intervention

☐ Documenting the plan of nursing care

Setting Priorities

Because nurses today are caring for a greater number of patients, and because those patients are more acutely ill, learning how to set priorities is vital to establishing a good plan of care. You must become skilled at differentiating between what is nice to do and what must be done, and learn to do what must be done before what is nice to do. However, the skill of setting priorities takes time to acquire because it depends upon your ability to view more than just individual problems: you must gain insight into the *entire picture* of all the problems at hand, and how they are affecting the *individuals* involved.

For example, normally if you had a patient who was having trouble breathing, you would correct this problem first. However, if in looking at the *whole picture*, you noted that the person was having trouble breathing because he was having an attack of anxiety, you would recognize that the first problem that should be resolved might be that of alleviating the anxiety so that breathing would be easier. Knowing the whole picture often changes how you assign priorities.

The activity of setting priorities occurs during both the initial planning phase and the implementation phase. During the *initial planning phase*, you need to assign priorities for setting forth the nursing care plan. During the *implementation phase*, you need to assign priorities on a day-to-day basis. This chapter will deal with setting priorities during the initial planning stage.

Setting priorities during the initial planning phase includes the following:

☐ Determining the problems that need *immediate attention* (i.e., life-threatening problems), and taking immediate appropriate action.

☐ Determining the nursing diagnoses that will be addressed on the nursing care plan (those diagnoses that are unusual or complex).

☐ Determining the collaborative problems that require physician's orders for diagnosis, monitoring, or treatment.

The following are basic principles that should be applied when assigning priorities, and suggested steps for setting priorities during the initial planning phase.

Basic Principles of Setting Priorities

☐ Priority ratings will be influenced by the following:

The Client's Own Perception of Priorities: Ask the person what he feels is important, and explain your rationale if you have to impose a different set of priorities.

The Overall Treatment Plan: For example, you may plan to have the person eat earlier than usual on the days he has a physical therapy treatment.

The Overall Health Status of the Client: For example, the nursing diagnosis of *Knowledge Deficit* may be given a high priority rating for a newly diagnosed diabetic if the person is generally healthy. However, this same problem would be given a low priority if the patient were too ill to learn.

The Presence of Potential Problems: For example, assisting a patient to stand immediately postoperatively to reduce the potential of falling takes priority over the patient's desire to stand on his own.

Rationale: Priority ratings will be influenced by viewing the *entire picture* of the problems and how they are affecting the individual's health status.

☐ Nurses and students should choose a method of assigning priority ratings, and use it consistently. For example, you may want to use Maslow's Hierarchy of Needs listed below.

Priority #1:   Problems interfering with physiological needs (*e.g.*, problems with respiration, circulation, nutrition, hydration, elimination, temperature regulation, physical comfort)

Priority #2:   Problems interfering with safety and security (*e.g.*, environmental hazards, fear)

Priority #3:   Problems interfering with love and belonging (*e.g.*, isolation or loss of a loved one)

Priority #4:   Problems interfering with self-esteem (*e.g.*, inability to wash hair, perform normal activities)

Priority #5:   Problems interfering with the ability to achieve personal goals

Rationale: Using the same method consistently will help you become systematic and comprehensive.

☐ Problems that are *contributing factors* to other problems should be resolved first. For example, if a person has joint pain and is not moving well, resolving the pain is likely to help him move better.

Rationale: The first step to resolving a problem is to remove or reduce its contributing factors. In the example above, if you try to help the patient move without resolving or reducing the problem of pain, you are unlikely to be successful.

Suggested Steps for Setting Priorities During the Initial Planning Stage

Step #1: Ask yourself, "Are there any problems here that need immediate attention? . . . What happens if I wait until later to attend to them?" As necessary, take immediate appropriate actions to initiate treatment (*e.g.*, notify the physician or head nurse, then initiate interventions to alleviate the problem).

Rationale: Identifying the consequences of what would happen if you wait until later to resolve a problem will help you determine what *must be done now.* Initiating a call for assistance *before* you continue to determine the rest of the plan of care expedites treatment of more severe problems.

Step #2: Having taken appropriate actions, list all the problems, and categorize them into two categories: *nursing diagnoses and collaborative problems.*

Rationale: Your responsibility for each of these types of problems is different. For nursing diagnoses you will be developing the plan of care independently. For collaborative problems, the plan of care will be determined by institutional standard protocols, procedures, policies, and by physician's orders.

Step #3: Study your list of collaborative problems, and determine whether you have physician's orders or standard protocols, policies, or procedures to direct their care and management.

Rationale: The physician should be notified if orders are necessary to direct the care and management of collaborative problems.

Step #4: Study your list of nursing diagnoses to determine which ones are unusual or complex, and address these on the care plan. (Ask yourself, "Which of these nursing diagnoses must be on the care plan?" . . . and, "What will happen if I don't put them on the care plan?")

Rationale: Routine nursing diagnoses should not go on the care plan. For example, if you worked in a nursing home, and your facility had a protocol for preventing *Impaired Skin Integrity* that was implemented for every patient, it would be redundant to address this on the care plan. Listing only the unusual or complex diagnoses on the care plan *highlights unusual problems* for other nurses and keeps you from spending time writing lengthy care plans that people are unlikely to read.

Setting Priorities
(*Suggested Answers on page 172*)

1. Fill in the blanks below:
   Setting priorities during the initial planning stage involves determining
   those problems that need (a) _____ attention, those problems that will
   be addressed on the (b) _____ _____ _____ ,and those problems
   that must be (c) _____ to the physician for diagnosis, monitoring, or
   treatment.

2. List four factors that may influence how you assign priorities to problems
   that you have identified.

   a.

   b.

   c.

   d.

3. Given a patient with the following problems, which problem *must* be
   treated immediately?

   a. _____ Diarrhea

   b. _____ Severe dyspnea

   c. _____ Altered Thought Processes related to unknown factors

4. Given a patient with the following problems, place an "N" in front of the
   problems that you *might* address on the care plan, and place an "R" in front
   of the problems that should be reported to the physician, or covered by
   hospital policies, procedures, or protocols.

   a. _____ Potential Fluid Volume Deficit related to increased metabolic
   needs

   b. _____ Potential blockage of Foley catheter related to passage of large
   clots

   c. _____ Management of heparin lock

   d. _____ Potential Impaired Skin Integrity related to fragile skin and
   immobility

   e. _____ Dehydration related to persistent vomiting

Giving Goal-Directed Care

Next to setting priorities, setting *realistic goals* is probably the most important
task of the planning phase. This is for the following reasons:

☐ Goals are the "measuring sticks" of the plan of care. (You will measure the
success of your plan by determining whether you achieved the goals that
you have set forth.)

☐ Goals direct your interventions. (How will you know what you are going to do, if you do not know what you are trying to accomplish?)

☐ Goals are motivating factors. (People usually do better if they are given a time frame for getting things done.)

Short-Term and Long-Term Goals

Giving goal-directed care includes setting both long-term and short-term goals. Short-term goals (STG) are those that can be met relatively quickly, often in less than a week. Long-term goals (LTG) are those that are to be achieved over a longer period of time, often weeks or months. Frequently, a nurse may set several short-term goals in order to reach a long-term goal. Table 4-1 gives some examples of short-term goals that may be stepping stones to long-term goals.

Long-term goals may also include goals that are ongoing (*i.e.*, goals that are to be accomplished every day). These types of long-term goals are usually stated by using the words "every day" or "will maintain." Note the examples below:

☐ "Louise will dress herself every morning."
☐ "Mr. Nathaniel will maintain a fluid intake of 2000 ml a day."

Many agencies use the abbreviation "LTG" to describe the *overall goal* of the plan of care. This type of long-term goal is also considered to be the "discharge goal" for the client. These long-term goals, or discharge goals,

Table 4-1. Examples of Short- and Long-Term Goals

Short-Term Goal	Long-Term Goal
"Mrs. Smith will demonstrate how to hold her newborn infant by tomorrow (6/9)."	"Mrs. Smith will demonstrate how to dress, feed, and bathe her newborn infant by discharge (6/13)."
"Mrs. Fox will turn and reposition herself from side to side every 2 hours."	"Mrs. Fox will maintain good skin integrity while she is on bedrest."
"Mr. Roberts will demonstrate how to change his colostomy bag within 2 days (by 7/7)."	"Mr. Roberts will demonstrate how to give complete colostomy care according to hospital standards by discharge (by 7/21)."
"Susie will walk with crutches with assistance by 3 days after surgery (by 7/28)."	"Susie will walk unassisted with a cane by discharge (by 8/10)."

should be clearly stated on the care plan so that the whole team knows that "this is what we are all working toward." For example, you may be caring for two women who are both in their seventies and have had surgery for a fractured hip. One of them may have an LTG of "returns to her husband and home, independently ambulatory with cane, capable of performing her usual activities of daily living," while the other woman's LTG may read "returns to nursing home and continued complete bedrest with healed fracture, good leg alignment, and without complications." Writing overall LTGs on the care plan is important so everyone who contributes to carrying out the plan is realistic and clear concerning what they expect the plan of care to accomplish.

Applying Nursing Standards When Setting Goals.   When you are establishing goals, it is necessary to apply accepted standards of nursing care (*i.e.*, your outcomes and plan of nursing care must reflect that you have set forth a plan that will achieve acceptable standards of care). Standards of care will be determined by the following:

□ **The Law:** Nurse practice acts, which delineate the scope of nursing and the ways in which nurses should practice, differ from state to state. You must be aware of your individual state practice acts.

□ **The American Nurses' Association (ANA):** The ANA has established standards that should be applied in all areas of nursing practice. They have also set standards for the specialty areas (*e.g.*, maternity, community health, rehabilitation).

□ **The Institution:** Each institution usually evolves its own unique set of standards that reflect the values and beliefs of the system (*i.e.*, the institution decides what objectives must be met in order to demonstrate optimum nursing care and then decides what interventions are necessary to accomplish the objectives). These objectives and interventions then become the standards that are set down in the policies and procedure manuals of the institution (see Fig. 4-1).

When you are setting client goals and planning nursing care you must apply the standards that are set forth by the law, the ANA, and the institution where you are working. ANA standards apply to all nurses everywhere and are applied throughout your nursing education. Individual state laws and institutional policies and procedures differ, so you must make yourself responsible for learning these as you move from institution to institution (*i.e.*, be sure to read policy and procedures manuals and become familiar with your state practice act).

Client-Centered Goals

Instead of writing nursing goals (*i.e.*, what the *nurse* aims to achieve), writing *client-centered goals* has been recognized as an efficient and effective method of writing goal statements. This is because client-centered goals focus upon

Standard of Nursing Care for Patients Admitted for Abdominal Surgery

Overall Goal: The individual will experience a safe, comfortable recovery from abdominal surgery with prevention of, and early detection and treatment of, possible complications as evidenced by the following:

1. Before and after surgery, the patient (and s/o, if appropriate) will be able to:

   — explain the type of surgery to be done in his/her own words
   — describe the preoperative and postoperative therapeutic plan of care and its rationale
   — relate the expected length of recuperation
   — voice concerns, anxieties, or fears and receive appropriate counseling/interventions as necessary
   — participate in measures to aid recovery and prevent complications

2. During the postoperative period, the nurse will document the following daily and prn:

   — vital signs with systems review (neurological, pulmonary, cardiac, circulatory, gastrointestinal, genitourinary, skin)
   — appearance of wound/dressings
   — color and amount of drainage/type of drains
   — intake and output
   — activity tolerance
   — comfort state, effectiveness of medication regimen, and nursing measures taken to enhance desired effects, or minimize side effects.
   — nursing actions taken when *early* signs and symptoms of possible complications of abdominal surgery become evident (*i.e.,* unstable vital signs, excessive drainage/bleeding, nonfunctioning drains or tubes, nonrelieved pain, excessive vomiting, abdominal distention, signs and symptoms of infection, deterioration in mental status, evidence of altered venous flow in lower extremities, diminished breath sounds and/or poor cough effort)

3. Before and after surgery, the nurse will document appropriate nursing diagnoses and individualized nursing approaches on the nursing care plan.

4. By discharge, the patient (and s/o, if appropriate) will be able to

   — relate plan of care and its rationale
   — participate actively in the plan of care
   — identify resources (personal/community) available if assistance in that care is necessary

Figure 4-1.   Sample hospital standard of care form for a specific collaborative problem. (Adapted from Standard of Nursing Care for Patients Admitted for Abdominal Surgery, Paoli Memorial Hospital, Paoli, Pennsylvania)

the *desired end result* of the plan of care: *that the client benefits from nursing care.* To be sure that you write client-centered goals, remember the following rule:

> **Rule:** The subject of a client-centered goal must be either the patient, or a part of the patient. (For example, "Chuck will ambulate three times a day in the room." "The skin will remain intact, free from signs of irritation.")

Below are some additional examples of client-centered goals.

> "Ms. Michaels will lose 5 lb in 3 weeks (by 7/31)."
> "Mrs. Matthews will walk unassisted with crutches by 2/6."
> "Mr. Daniels will demonstrate sterile injection technique by 9/18."

Goals vs. Outcomes

The terms *goals, outcomes,* and *objectives* are often used interchangeably because they are all statements of what is expected to be accomplished by a certain time. Some authors view goals and objectives as being more general descriptions, and outcomes as being more specific. More recently, it has been suggested to use broad goals or objectives *together with specific outcomes* so that the goal statement clearly describes the data that is expected to be observed that will demonstrate that the goal has been achieved. For example, you may have a broad goal or objective of "will demonstrate effective airway clearance," and be required to list exactly what you expect to observe or hear (outcome data) that will tell you that the individual is able to clear his airway. In this situation, your goal statement would look like this:

> The client will demonstrate effective airway clearance as evidenced by clear lungs, ability to bring forth sputum with cough, and absence of fever.

The first part of the statement is the *broad goal,* and the second part of the statement (after the "as evidenced by") are the *outcomes,* which describe the *specific data* that will tell you that the broad goal has been achieved. Remember the following rule:

> **Rule:** The terms *goals, objectives,* and *outcomes* are often used interchangeably, with outcomes usually being more specific. When you need to be *very specific* in writing a goal statement, state the broad goal, add "as evidenced by," and list the data (outcomes) that will tell you that the patient has achieved the goal. (*Example:* Will demonstrate knowledge of medication regimen as evidenced by ability to relate drug names, doses, times, purpose, and side effects.)

Determining Goals (Outcomes) from Nursing Diagnoses

For every nursing diagnosis that you list on the nursing care plan, you must identify a *client-centered goal* that would demonstrate an improvement or resolution of the nursing diagnosis. *Goal statements are derived directly from the nursing diagnoses* that you have identified. This means that if your diagnoses are incorrect, your goals are likely to be inappropriate.

Sometimes you will find that you decide to write more than one goal for a given problem. In these cases, the goals will probably relate to the etiology of the problem rather than to the problem itself. It is important that *at least one* of the goals demonstrates a direct resolution of, or improvement in, the nursing diagnosis. Note the following example:

> **Nursing Diagnosis:** *Altered Nutrition: More Than Body Requirements related to poor eating habits and minimal physical activity*
> *Goal #1:* Client will describe daily menus that demonstrate healthy meal choices and decreased intake of empty calories. (This goal relates to the problem of "poor eating habits," which is a causative factor.)
> *Goal #2:* Client will attend daily exercise classes. (This goal relates to the problem of "minimal physical activity," which is a causative factor.)
> *Goal #3:* Client will lose 1 lb per week beginning 10/25 until she weighs between 135 and 145 lb. (This goal demonstrates a *direct resolution* of the problem of *Altered Nutrition: More Than Body Requirements*.)

Remember the following rule:

Rule: Be sure that at least one of the goals that you set demonstrates a direct resolution of or improvement in the nursing diagnosis.

Study the steps for deriving goals from nursing diagnoses below.

1. Look at the first clause of the nursing diagnosis or problem statement (*i.e.*, the word or words before "related to").

   EXAMPLE: First Clause

   Potential Inpaired Skin Integrity related to immobility

2. Now *restate the first clause* in a goal statement that would describe an improvement in or absence of the problem.

   EXAMPLE: The client will demonstrate no signs of skin irritation or breakdown.

Table 4-2 lists several examples of outcomes derived from nursing diagnoses that have been identified during a nursing assessment.

Rules for Stating Client Outcomes/Goals from Nursing Diagnoses.   As already discussed, client outcome statements must be specific. They must state *what*

Table 4-2. Client Outcomes (Goals) Derived from Nursing Diagnoses

Nursing Diagnosis	Corresponding Client Outcome (Goal)
Altered Nutrition: Less Than Body Requirements	The client will demonstrate normal nutritional state as evidenced by weight of 120–130 lbs, and record of eating balanced meals with few snacks every day.
Ineffective Individual Coping	The client will demonstrate and relate effective coping as evidenced by self report of coping better, and ability to demonstrate good problem-solving.
Constipation	The client will demonstrate normal bowel function as evidenced by having a normal stool once or twice daily and by statements of feeling as though bowels are moving well.

is to be done, *who* is to do it, *when* they are to do it, *how* they are to do it, *where* they are to do it, and *how well* they are to do it. To ensure that outcomes are specific, there are rules for writing outcome statements. Each goal or outcome statement must have the components listed below:

Subject: *Who* is the person expected to achieve the goal?

Verb: *What actions* must the person do to achieve the goal?

Condition: *Under what circumstances* is the person to perform the actions?

Criteria: *How well* is the person to perform the action?

Specific Time: *When* is the person expected to perform the action?

Example: Mr. Smith will walk with a cane at least to the end of the hall and back this afternoon.

Subject: Mr. Smith

Verb: will walk

Condition: with a cane

Criteria: at least to the end of the hall and back

Time: this afternoon.

Making sure that the goal statement has all five of these components ensures a very specific statement that can later be evaluated to see how well the patient has achieved the established goal.

"Fine Tuning" Outcome Statements.   Because client outcome statements deal with describing exactly what a patient must be able to *do*, it is important that you use clear and specific verbs to descibe what is to be done. For example, a nurse who wants the patient to understand how to use sterile technique may be tempted to write an outcome statement such as, "The patient will understand how to use sterile technique." However, this statement would be too vague. You must ask yourself, "*How* will I *know* if he understands?" The only way that you can be sure if he does indeed understand is if he actually verbalizes or demonstrates how to use sterile technique. Verbs used in writing outcome statements must be verbs that are *measurable* (*i.e.*, verbs that describe the exact behavior that you expect to *see* or *hear*). Below are some examples of verbs that are measurable and verbs that are nonmeasurable. *When writing client outcomes, avoid using the verbs listed in the nonmeasurable columns.*

Measurable Verbs

identify	hold	exercise
describe	demonstrate	communicate
perform	share	cough
relate	express	walk
state	has an increase in	stand
list	has a decrease in	sit
verbalize	has an absence of	discuss

Nonmeasurable Verbs

know	think
understand	accept
appreciate	feel

There are many things to consider when establishing goals. The following guidelines are suggested to help you set client goals.

☐ *Guidelines*   *Establishing Client Goals/Outcomes from Nursing Diagnoses*

☐ Be realistic in establishing goals. Be sure to consider the following:

Growth and development

Behavioral patterns of the individual

Physical health state

Available human and material resources

Other planned therapies for the client

The time frame in which the client may be expected to achieve an expected outcome

☐ Whenever possible, set goals mutually with the client and others involved in his healthcare (*e.g.*, family, other healthcare workers) to ensure that the goals are congruent with other planned therapies.

☐ Establish both short- and long-term goals (the short-term goals can be used as steps toward meeting the long-term goal).

☐ Be sure that the client goals that you write describe a client behavior or action that demonstrates the desired improvement or resolution of the problems identified by the nursing diagnoses.

☐ Follow the rules for writing goal statements.

☐ Use measurable, observable verbs to describe the desired actions or behaviors that you expect to see.

☐ Identify only one behavior per outcome. If you need to write two behaviors, write two outcomes.

EXAMPLE:

Wrong: Client will discuss the role of insulin in carbohydrate metabolism and give his own insulin.

Right: Client will discuss the role of insulin in carbohydrate metabolism. Client will give his own insulin.

☐ Be sure that the subject of your outcome statement is the client (or family) or some part of the client.

EXAMPLES:

Bob will rest lying down for a half hour after meals.
The *skin* around the incision will remain clean and dry at all times.

☐ Be sure that your outcomes reflect the accepted standards of the ANA, your state practice act, and the institution where you are working.

☐ *Practice Session*   *Writing Client Goals/Outcomes from Nursing Diagnoses*
(Suggested Answers on page 173)

1. List at least five measurable verbs.

2. Choose the client goal statements that are written correctly below. Identify what is wrong with the statements that are written incorrectly.

   a. John will know the basic four food groups by 1/4.

b. Mrs. Smith will demonstrate how to use her walker by Saturday.

c. Mr. Jones will improve his appetite by 1/6.

d. Jane will list the equipment needed to change sterile dressings by 2/2.

e. Susan will walk independently in the hall after surgery.

f. Mrs. Baylis will understand the importance of maintaining a salt-free diet.

g. June will ambulate to the bathroom with the use of her cane by 3/4.

h. Mrs. Smith will appreciate the importance of childproofing her home.

i. Janet will lose 5 lb by 1/9.

j. Mr. Collins will feel less pain by Thursday.

3. For each diagnosis or problem below, write an appropriate client outcome. Be sure that each client outcome that you write has all of the necessary components.

   a. Constipation related to insufficient roughage intake in diet

   b. Altered Oral Mucous Membrane related to poor oral hygiene

   c. Potential Impaired Skin Integrity related to draining abdominal incision

   d. Impaired Verbal Communication related to inability to speak English

   e. Spiritual Distress related to inability to attend daily Mass

   f. Self-Care Deficit: Feeding related to weakness of both hands

   g. Potential Ineffective Airway Clearance related to smoking

   h. Altered Nutrition: Less Than Body Requirements related to loss of appetite

i. Sleep Pattern Disturbance related to need for frequent treatments and assessment of vital signs

j. Urge Incontinence related to unknown factors

Affective, Cognitive, and Psychomotor Outcomes/Objectives. Expected outcomes can be classified into three domains: cognitive, affective, and psychomotor. Below is a description of each of the domains.

☐ **Cognitive Domain:** Outcomes that are associated with acquired knowledge or intellectual abilities (*e.g.*, learning the signs and symptoms of diabetic shock)

☐ **Psychomotor Domain:** Outcomes that deal with developing motor skills (*e.g.*, mastering how to walk with crutches)

☐ **Affective Domain:** Outcomes that are associated with changes in attitudes, feelings, or values (*e.g.*, deciding that old eating habits need to be changed)

Display 4-1 lists verbs that are representative of each domain.

Correctly identifying the domains of the client outcomes is useful for planning nursing strategies. Many beginning nurses assume that the only strategies that are necessary are those that promote new knowledge or skills and forget to be concerned with the need for a new set of values. For example, it could be useless to instruct a client how to stick to a diabetic diet if he did not value the importance of being on the diet in the first place. Often more than one domain may be involved in the achievement of one outcome. For example,

Display 4-1. Verbs Representative of the Three Domains		
Cognitive	**Affective**	**Psychomotor**
teach	express	demonstrate
discuss	share	practice
identify	listen	perform
describe	communicate	walk
list	relate	administer
explore		give

you may have identified the expected outcome of "Mrs. Laird will prepare three balanced meals for her children." In order to achieve this outcome, Mrs. Laird will have to achieve outcomes in all three domains. She will have to:

☐ State the foods that should be included in a balanced diet (cognitive)

☐ Share her feelings concerning being responsible for her children's nutrition (affective)

☐ Demonstrate cooking and serving the meal (psychomotor)

☐ *Practice Session*   *Domains of Expected Outcomes*
(Suggested Answers on page 174)

1. Identify whether each of the expected outcomes listed below is in the affective, cognitive, or psychomotor domain. (Remember, there may be more than one domain for each outcome.)

    a. Mrs. Resh will demonstrate how to prepare and sterilize her baby's formula.

    b. Becky will discuss the importance of sterilization.

    c. Judy will relate her feelings concerning going home.

    d. Mrs. Ballard will discuss the relationship between blood sugar levels and food.

    e. Connie will administer her own insulin according to the results of her morning blood sugar readings.

    f. Mr. Roberts will walk the length of the hall with a cane.

    g. Mrs. Bell will verbalize when she is worried or concerned.

    h. Debbie will demonstrate how to perform postural drainage.

    i. Matt will verbalize the signs and symptoms of hypoglycemia.

    j. Jimmy will eat a balanced breakfast every morning.

2. Once you have identified the domains of the expected outcomes in the above examples, write one or two activities that would help the client to achieve the outcome. (Note the example below.)

    EXAMPLE:

    Sample outcome: Mrs. Jones will be able to dress herself without assistance by 7/4.
    Domain: Psychomotor
    Activities: Practice buttoning buttons and tying shoes on 7/1 and 7/2.
    Practice putting on blouse, skirt, shoes, and socks on 7/3.
    Demonstrate dressing herself on 7/4.

Determining Goals for Collaborative Problems

The *overall goals of nursing* for all collaborative problems are the following, no matter what the problem:

☐ To detect and report early signs and symptoms of potential complications of the collaborative problem

☐ To implement preventive and corrective nursing interventions ordered by the physician (or by standards, protocols, procedures, and policies)

In most facilities, goals for collaborative problems are not documented other than in standards, protocols, procedures, and policy manuals (in the form of objectives or overall goals). Take a moment to study Figure 4-1 on page 97, which gives an example of a standard that guides the nursing care of the collaborative problem of abdominal surgery. You will note that the overall goal for this problem is stated at the beginning of the standard, in the form of a client-centered goal. Also note that #2 in the standard states, "the nurse will document. . . . " (instead of, "the nurse will monitor . . . "). This is because the only way anyone will be able to determine whether the goal of monitoring for potential complications and reporting early signs and symptoms has been met is *by checking the documentation. You* may know that you met your goal of reporting signs and symptoms of potential complications and implementing preventive and corrective interventions as ordered by the physician, but if you do not document all this, *only you can be sure.*

Let me clarify further. Suppose you have the *collaborative problem* of an intravenous line, and you have the overall goal of "monitoring for early detection and treatment of potential complications of the IV." The only way anyone will know if you have met this goal is by checking your documentation and determining whether you actually assessed the patient at specific intervals, and acted appropriately to facilitate treatment when the signs and symptoms became evident. (You see, the patient *may never have exhibited* signs and symptoms of potential complications, but how does anyone know that *you met the goal of looking for them,* if you do not document it?) This is why you will find an emphasis on documentation in standards, policies, protocols, and procedure manuals.*

Determining Nursing Interventions

Nursing interventions are specific nursing activities or actions that a nurse must perform to prevent complications, provide for comfort (physical, psychological, and spiritual), and promote, maintain, and restore health. The activ-

---

* Documentation will be discussed in detail later in this chapter, and in Chapter 5, Implementation.

ities listed below are interventions that nurses are likely to identify when planning for comprehensive patient care.

☐ Performing nursing assessments to identify new problems and to determine the status of existing problems

☐ Performing patient teaching to help clients gain new knowledge concerning their own health

☐ Counseling clients to make decisions about their own healthcare

☐ Consulting with and referring to other healthcare professionals to obtain appropriate direction

☐ Performing specific treatment actions to remove, reduce, or resolve health problems

☐ Assisting clients to perform activities themselves

Let's consider the nurse's role of assessing, teaching, counseling, and consulting when providing for patient care.

Nursing Assessment as an Intervention

Performing a focus assessment of identified problems is a nursing intervention that should be employed before performing any other intervention. For example, if you use the nursing diagnosis of *Fluid Volume Deficit related to insufficient fluid intake,* you must assess how much the person has actually had to drink before you encourage him to drink more. It could be possible that he has overcompensated and is now drinking more than he should. Blindly continuing nursing interventions without performing a focus assessment of the problem can create *new* problems and be detrimental to the individual's health.

Teaching as an Intervention

Teaching is an intervention that is common to many problems. It may be a specific intervention (such as teaching an individual to give his own injection) or it may be an adjunct intervention (such as explaining the rationale for coughing and deep breathing while you are assisting the patient to cough and breathe deeply). Teaching is a vital nursing intervention that should be implemented at every opportunity. The following guidelines are suggested to help you in planning patient teaching.

☐ *Guidelines*   *Planning Patient Teaching*

☐ Always assess readiness to learn and previous knowledge before you begin a teaching plan.

☐ Set goals with the client so that both of you know what you are aiming to teach (*e.g.*, "Let's see if by this afternoon you can describe menus that would contain three balanced meals").

☐ Use terminology that the client understands.

☐ Encourage the client to ask questions and verbalize his understanding of what is being taught (*e.g.*, by stating, "I want you to feel free to ask questions no matter how stupid you think they are. We all feel dumb from time to time, so don't feel you are the only one. Your questions are important, no matter how small.").

☐ Find ways to include the family and significant others in the teaching session (when appropriate).

☐ Plan for a quiet private environment that is conducive to learning.

☐ Identify active learning experiences (*i.e.*, use examples, simulations, games, and audiovisuals when appropriate).

☐ Plan to pace learning. Do not give too much information at one time (*i.e.*, progress at the individual's learning pace).

☐ Allow time to discuss progress (*e.g.*, ask the patient how he feels he is progressing and let him know how you feel he is progressing).

☐ Include time for summarizing what has been taught (*e.g.*, at the beginning of a session and at the end of a session).

Counseling as an Intervention

Counseling clients to help them make necessary changes or adjustments in their lives or to help them make choices about their healthcare is an important nursing activity. Counseling includes using teaching techniques to help the patient acquire the necessary knowledge to make decisions about his own healthcare. It also includes offering emotional and psychological support to the individual and his family as they seek to adjust to new circumstances of living. Through the use of teaching techniques and therapeutic communication, a nurse can offer valuable psychological and intellectual support and can reduce the level of stress for both the patient and family.

Consulting and Referring as an Intervention

Whenever the client's problems require more than independent nursing interventions, part of the nursing plan for interventions must be that of consulting with or referring to the appropriate healthcare professional. For example, if the client states that he has trouble swallowing pills, a nurse might consult with the pharmacist to determine if there is a better method of giving the medications. If a person has a poor nutritional intake because he dislikes hospital food, the nurse should refer the problem to the hospital dietitian so that perhaps different meals can be served. Nurses must always refer medical problems and complications to physicians so that collaborative nursing interventions can be determined.

Incorporating Physicians' Orders

A comprehensive plan of care incorporates physicians' orders as well as nursing orders (*i.e.*, physicians' orders must always be checked *before* planning nursing interventions). This is because physicians' orders may direct care of collaborative problems, and *are likely to affect how you plan care for nursing diagnoses*. For example, you may have identified the nursing diagnosis of *Activity Intolerance*. You would be unable to determine whether you could actually treat this problem or how you would treat this problem unless you knew what activities were allowed by the physician. Before you determine interventions, you should routinely check for orders concerning the following:

☐ Diet/activity restrictions
☐ Frequency of recording of vital signs, or other special assessment (*e.g.*, neuro checks)
☐ Medications/intravenous fluids
☐ Treatments/diagnostic studies

Physicians' orders often include specific nursing interventions that will prevent or correct potential complications. Examples of these are the following:

☐ Irrigating a nasogastric tube or Foley catheter to prevent it from becoming blocked by clots or sediment
☐ Maintaining suction for drainage tubes to facilitate drainage
☐ Administering anticoagulants to prevent thrombus formation
☐ Administering intravenous fluids to prevent dehydration or electrolyte imbalance

Physician's orders may also modify or complement routine interventions for collaborative problems listed on standards, protocols, policies, and procedures. If the interventions contradict normal policies, you should check with the physician whether he was aware of the policies. If no change is made, and the orders contradict normal policies, you should report this to the head nurse or supervisor.

In the hospital setting, physicians' orders are usually transcribed to two places:

☐ Medication and IV orders are transcribed to medication and IV record forms*

---

* These forms vary from institution to institution, although they have basically the same information.

☐ Treatments, diagnostic studies, and other orders are transcribed to the "treatment kardex"*

Just as the nursing care plan is used as a guide to direct care for nursing diagnoses, the above two types of records are *essential to directing care for medical and collaborative problems.*

How physicians' orders for nursing interventions are transcribed to the plan of care may vary from institution to institution. However, your responsibility in transcribing the orders is the same everywhere. Before you transcribe an order you should be sure you know why it is to be done. When you transcribe the order, you should be sure that both the physician and you are clear about the following:

☐ Exactly what intervention is to be done
☐ Exactly how the intervention is to be done
☐ Exactly when and how often it is to be done
☐ Exactly how much, how often, for how long, and by what route (in the case of medications or intravenous fluids)

If the physician has not been clear about any of the above information, you should clarify the order before transcribing it.†

Determining Nursing Interventions For Nursing Diagnoses

Determining nursing interventions for specific nursing diagnoses involves determining the nursing actions or activities that will achieve the established expected outcomes. That is, what are you going to do to reduce or resolve each of the nursing diagnoses that you have identified?

There are three questions that are important when determining nursing interventions for nursing diagnoses.

1. What is the cause (etiology) of the problem?
2. What can be done to eliminate or minimize the cause?
3. How can I help the client achieve the expected outcomes?

In order to determine nursing interventions for a potential or actual nursing diagnosis, you must identify its etiology and decide what can be done to reduce or eliminate it. How to identify the etiology of nursing diagnoses was discussed in Chapter 3 (see Determining the Etiology of Nursing Diagnoses). You should also remember from Chapter 3 that the etiology is found in the second clause of the problem statement for the nursing diagnosis (*i.e.*, after

---

* Kardexes are usually placed in a flip-chart device for quick retrieval of information.
† Recommended reading: Cushing, M. (1986) Who transcribed that order? *Am. J Nurs.* (10):1107–1108.

"related to"). Look at the example problem statement for *Fluid Volume Deficit related to insufficient fluid intake.*

Second Clause
↓

Fluid Volume Deficit related to insufficient fluid intake

Once you have determined the cause or contributing factors of the actual or potential nursing diagnosis, you must determine nursing interventions that would either eliminate the factors or minimize their effects. For example, if you identify the actual or potential diagnosis of *Impaired Skin Integrity related to prescribed bedrest,* you should determine interventions that would reduce the effect of the prescribed bedrest. That is, you would plan a regimen of turning the patient from side to side and gently massaging areas that may receive more pressure than usual (*e.g.*, coccyx). If the diagnosis is described as a *potential* diagnosis, you would also have to establish a regimen of frequent focus assessments to be sure that the potential diagnosis has not become an *actual* diagnosis. If the diagnosis is described as an actual diagnosis, you should also plan to perform frequent focus assessments of the clinical manifestations of the diagnosis to monitor the status of the problem. For example, suppose you identified the actual nursing diagnosis of *Impaired Skin Integrity related to prescribed bedrest as manifested by an area of red, scaly dry skin around the coccyx 2 inches in diameter.* You may plan to assess the area around the coccyx every 2 hours to assess for improvement or deterioration in the signs and symptoms.

If you identify a *possible* nursing diagnosis, the interventions that you would prescribe would be those that would lead you to gain more information to help you to decide if the diagnosis is indeed present. For example, if you have identified the possible diagnosis of *Possible Ineffective Individual Coping,* you would prescribe interventions such as "Provide time for discussing how this individual feels that he is coping with his current problems."

Display 4-2 summarizes how to determine nursing interventions for actual, potential, and possible nursing diagnosis.

Considering Expected Outcomes to "Fine Tune" Nursing Interventions. To "fine tune" nursing interventions, the expected outcomes of the plan of care should be considered as well as the etiology of the problem. For example, consider the nursing diagnosis of *Fluid Volume Deficit related to insufficient fluid intake.* Studying the etiology should lead you to identify the nursing intervention of "increase fluid intake." Considering the expected outcome of "will demonstrate adequate hydration as evidenced by absence of signs of dehydration and fluid intake of at least 2000 cc/day" will help you determine exactly how much fluid the person has to drink in order to prevent, reduce, or eliminate the problem. Considering both the etiology and the expected outcome will help

Display 4-2. How to Determine Nursing Interventions for Actual, Potential, and Possible Nursing Diagnoses

For an Actual Nursing Diagnosis:

1. Study the etiology (clause after "related to") and identify interventions that would reduce or remove the contributing factors.
2. Plan a regimen to perform frequent focus assessments of the clinical manifestations to monitor the status of the signs and symptoms of the problem.

For a Potential Nursing Diagnosis:

1. Study the etiology and identify interventions that would reduce or remove the contributing factors.
2. Plan a regimen to perform frequent focus assessments to be sure that clinical manifestations have not appeared that would change the status of the diagnosis from potential to actual.

For a Possible Nursing Diagnosis:

Identify methods of collecting more data about the possible diagnosis to determine if any of the clinical manifestations or common contributing factors of the diagnosis are indeed present.

you to determine exactly what nursing actions will help this particular patient achieve the expected outcomes.

The following guidelines are suggested to assist you in determining nursing interventions for nursing diagnoses.

☐ *Guidelines*   *Planning Nursing Interventions for Nursing Diagnoses*

☐ Identify focus assessments of the problem before determining appropriate nursing interventions.

☐ Look for interventions that will reduce or eliminate the etiology (cause) of the problem.

☐ Consider the expected outcome to be sure that your interventions are specific for that particular patient.

☐ Identify the strengths of the client and his family that can be encouraged so that they can participate in correcting the problem.

☐ Individualize nursing actions. What may work for one person may not for another.

☐ Be realistic. Nursing interventions should

   Consider the patient's limitations/preferences

   Consider the developmental age of the client

Be within the knowledge and capabilities of the nurse

Be congruent with other therapies

Provide safe and therapeutic environment

Utilize appropriate resources

☐ Utilize scientific rationale as a basis for your actions (know the rationale for the interventions you choose).

☐ Create opportunities for teaching and learning whenever possible (*e.g.*, teach the patient the reasons for the nursing actions that you have chosen).

☐ Consult other professionals when indicated (*e.g.*, dietitian).

☐ *Practice Session*   *Determining Nursing Interventions for Nursing Diagnoses*
(Suggested Answers on page 175)

For each of the nursing diagnoses and goals (outcome criteria) listed below, list some possible nursing interventions that would help the client to reach the set goal.

1. **Nursing Diagnosis:** *Potential Impaired Skin Integrity related to prescribed bedrest*

   Outcome Criteria: Client will maintain good skin integrity while he is on bedrest.

   List appropriate nursing interventions:

2. **Nursing Diagnosis:** *Potential Ineffective Airway Clearance related to thoracic incision pain*

   Outcome Criteria: Client will demonstrate effective coughing and deep breathing every 2 hours for the first day after surgery.

   List appropriate nursing interventions:

3. **Nursing Diagnosis:** *Constipation related to insufficient exercise and inadequate fluid and roughage intake*

   Outcome Criteria: Client will have daily soft bowel movements.

   List appropriate nursing interventions:

4. **Nursing Diagnosis:** *Potential Infection related to new incision*

   Outcome Criteria: Incision will show no signs of infection (redness, swelling, drainage). Incision will be protected from microbial invasion by a clean, dry dressing at all times.

   List appropriate nursing interventions:

5. **Nursing Diagnosis:** *Powerlessness related to hospitalization*

   Outcome Criteria: Client will verbalize his feelings concerning being placed in the position of powerlessness while in the hospital. Client will be able to verbalize those things that he feels he should be allowed to control. Client will control his own care as much as possible.

   List appropriate nursing interventions.

Determining Nursing Interventions for Collaborative Problems

Nursing interventions for collaborative problems include the following:

☐ Performing frequent assessments to monitor the status of the patient and to detect early signs and symptoms of pathophysiologic complications. (*Exam-*

ple: Assessing lung sounds every two hours when there is a possibility of developing congestive heart failure.)

☐ Alerting the physician when early signs and symptoms of potential pathophysiologic complications are suspected. (*Example:* Contacting the physician when a patient's urine output has dropped to less than 30 cc/hr.)

☐ Performing preventive and corrective nursing actions as ordered by the physician. (*Example:* A physician may write "irrigate the nasogastric tube every 2 hours.")

☐ Performing nursing actions as described in standard policy and procedure manuals. (*Example:* Providing special Foley catheter care once every shift.)

Monitoring to Detect Potential Complications.   Monitoring to detect potential complications takes a high level of theoretical and practical knowledge. The following guidelines are suggested to help you determine exactly how you would monitor a given collaborative problem.

☐ *Guidelines*   *Monitoring to Detect Potential Complications*

1. Determine a baseline (*i.e.*, assess the current status of the problem in this specific situation).

EXAMPLE:

If you are monitoring the status of a patient on a respirator and his blood gases have been consistently abnormal, consult with the physician or nurse specialist to determine the current acceptable arterial blood gases for this specific patient. What may be normal for this individual in this situation may be abnormal for another in a similar situation.

2. Determine exactly *what* is to be assessed, and *how* and *when* it is to be assessed.

EXAMPLE:

All central venous pressure readings will be taken every hour with the patient flat in bed.

3. Determine early signs and symptoms of potential complications.

EXAMPLE:

Potential complication: hypovolemia. Early signs and symptoms would be increasing heart rate, drop in blood pressure, drop in urine output, and changes in mental status. (You would assess for the presence of any of these signs and symptoms.)

4. Determine the exact method of recording assessment findings for problem.

EXAMPLE:

Keep a neurological assessment flow sheet that clearly describes neurological status.

5. Determine what assessment findings would indicate possible deterioration in the patient's condition and would require you to notify the physician.

EXAMPLE:

The physician should be notified if the patient has less than 30 ml of urine output for 2 consecutive hours.

□ *Practice Session*   *Monitoring to Detect Potential Complications*
(Suggested Answers on page 176)

For each of the collaborative problems below, identify potential complications and determine how, and how often, you would plan to monitor for the problems. (You may need to use an additional resource, such as a medical-surgical textbook, for this section.)

1. Intravenous infusion at 25 cc/hr.
   Potential Complications:

   Plan for monitoring to detect potential complications:

2. Insulin-dependent diabetes.
   Potential Complications:

   Plan for monitoring to detect potential complications:

3. Foley catheter.
   Potential Complications:

   Plan for monitoring to detect potential complications:

Using Standardized Care Plan Guides

Establishing goals and determining nursing interventions can be difficult for beginning nurses. However, today's nurses have an additional tool to help them in this complex task: the standardized care plan. As nurses have become more adept at researching and using the nursing process, they have begun to generate standard care plans that can be used as guides when identifying client outcomes and nursing interventions for certain situations. These standard care plans usually identify the common problems that are often seen with a given diagnosis. Standard care plans are now available from several different sources:

Institutional Care Plans. Many institutions maintain standard care plans on each unit. These care plans incorporate client outcomes and nursing interventions according to the unique standards of the institution.

Computerized Care Plans. These care plans can be broadly based on national standards but are often adapted specifically for a given institution.

Care Plans Printed in Books. Many books incorporate care plans that can be considered to be standard for a given medical or nursing diagnosis. Some are even written specifically with the intention of offering suggested standard care plans for nurses.

All of the above can be valuable tools in helping you to establish a comprehensive, individualized plan of nursing care that clearly describes client outcomes and pertinent nursing interventions. However, you must be sure that you use these standard care plans as they are intended to be used. *They are to be used as a guide, not as a crutch.* When used correctly, suggested care plan guides can provide the nurse with some basic information as she starts the care planning process. Using care plan guides helps to make the beginning work of care planning easier. Having this beginning work made easier helps to free the nurse to devote her time and creative energy to providing an individualized plan of care. You must carefully analyze the suggested care plan to determine what things are appropriate for your specific patient. Suggested standard care plans should always be used as a beginning, and never as an end. They should always be considered as beginning guides, never as set plans. Blindly using suggested care plans can be detrimental for your patient because it will be rare that all of your patient's specific problems will be addressed by one suggested care plan. Students and new graduates may find them to be valuable tools for learning, but they must be aware that *if they are used alone they can retard growth.* (Imagine if you only knew how to add, subtract, multiply, and divide by using a calculator!)

The following guidelines are suggested to help you to use standardized care plans to write *individualized client outcomes* and *individualized nursing interventions.*

Individualizing Standard Care Plans

☐ Use only appropriate sources for your care plan guide. Ask yourself the following:

1. Is this standard care plan approved (or accepted) by the particular institution (or school) with which you are working? (Students and beginning nurses should check with their instructor or staff development nurse before using a standard care plan as a guide.)

2. Does the standard care plan source cite bibliographic information to validate its resources?

3. Is the standard care plan congruent with the standards of care set forth by the law, the ANA, and the institution where you are working?

☐ To reduce temptation to use a standard care plan blindly, follow the steps below:

1. Always perform a complete nursing assessment and identify problems *yourself* first.

2. Once you have identified some problems yourself, check with the standard care plan to see if you have missed any of the problems that are associated with the ones that you have already diagnosed.

3. Assess your patient for the presence of these problems.

4. List all the problems that you have identified, and establish expected outcomes (goals). You may want to compare your goals with the goals suggested by the standard care plan, but remember: Goals must be highly specific and individualized.

5. Determine some nursing interventions *yourself* first.

6. Compare the interventions that you have identified with the interventions suggested by the standard care plan, and add any interventions that are appropriate for your patient. Delete interventions that are not appropriate.

Determining Nursing Orders

Once you have determined the nursing interventions that you will employ in giving nursing care, you will need to write nursing orders so that all nurses caring for that particular patient will have clear instructions for implementing the plan of care. Because client teaching and client assessment should be employed as adjunct interventions to every nursing action, you should consider the following when writing nursing orders:

☐ What to look for (assessment)

☐ What to do

☐ What to teach

☐ What to document

For example, suppose you were caring for a patient who had a hernia repair, and you had identified *Potential Ineffective Airway Clearance related to smoking.* You probably would plan to assist him with breathing and coughing exercises the first few days after surgery. Your orders for this situation may look like this:

1. Assess for rales/rhonchi/increased mucus production every 4 hours.
2. Assist the person to perform coughing and breathing exercises with pillow and hand over incision for support every 4 hours.
3. Reinforce (teach) the person the importance of coughing and deep breathing.
4. Document lung sounds and sputum production once a shift.

Nursing orders may not always need to describe assessment, teaching, and documentation, as well as the activity to be performed, but if you routinely consider whether you need to write orders for assessing, doing, teaching, and documenting, you are more likely to write comprehensive nursing orders that encompass more than just the activity to be performed.

"Fine Tuning" Nursing Orders.   Nursing orders must be specific and clear. They should include the following:

Date: The date the order was written

Verb: Action to be performed

Subject: Who is to do it

Descriptive Phrase: How, when, where, how often, how long, how much

Signature: Whoever wrote the order should sign it.

EXAMPLE:

4/29/89   Assist Chelsey* to sit on the side of the bed for 10 minutes t.i.d.
                                                                                M. Riley RN

If you added the dimensions of assessing, teaching, and documenting, the orders might look like this:

4/29/89   Assist to sit on side of bed t.i.d. for 10 minutes.

1. Monitor for dizziness or fatigue.
2. Reinforce the importance of gradual increase in activity level.
3. Document pulse rate before and after activity.
                                                                                M. Riley RN

Table 4-3 shows examples of nursing actions with corresponding nursing orders.

* The patient's name may be omitted, since it is understood (*e.g.,* "Assist to sit. . . . ")

**Table 4-3. Nursing Actions with Corresponding
Nursing Orders**

Nursing Action	Nursing Orders
Ambulate patient.	Ambulate patient the length of the hall using the walker three times a day.
Maintain caloric intake of 3,000 calories/day.	Consult dietitian to plan meals and snacks. Encourage patient to complete all his meals. Offer between-meal milkshakes (likes chocolate and strawberry) t.i.d. Have the patient keep a daily record of food eaten.
Provide for periods of uninterrupted rest.	Do not awaken from 12 MN to 7 AM— allow to rest from 1 PM to 3 PM (no visitors).

☐ *Practice Session*   *Writing Nursing Orders*
(*Suggested Answers on page 176*)

For each nursing intervention listed below, write appropriate nursing orders.

1. Maintain a program of turning from side to side.

2. Force fluids to 3000 ml/day.

3. Encourage patient to express her feelings.

4. Promote daily bowel elimination.

5. Get patient out of bed b.i.d.

Documenting the Nursing Care Plan

While physicians' orders and hospital standards and procedures set forth the medical treatment plan, *the nursing care plan focuses on nursing diagnoses.** When you are documenting a plan of care, you should keep in mind that your final product (the nursing care plan) will serve three purposes:

☐ It will direct nursing care.

☐ It will direct documentation.

☐ It will serve as the only written record that proves that a thoughtful, individualized *nursing* plan has been set forth, which will later be used as a tool for evaluation.

To fulfill its purpose, each care plan should include the following components:

☐ A brief client profile (name, age, height, weight, reason for seeking health-care, and any other pertinent information)

☐ Long-term overall discharge goal

☐ Nursing diagnoses and corresponding expected outcomes

☐ Specific nursing orders

☐ A space for evaluative comments (progress reports)

Forms for Documenting Care Plans

Forms for and methods of documenting care plans vary from institution to institution because they must be tailor-made to meet the needs of the nurses and clients in each unique setting. You will have to familiarize yourself with the methods used by the institution in which you will be working. If you are a student, you should expect that your care plans may be required to be detailed and comprehensive, addressing all aspects of the patient's care. However, care plans that are actually used in the practice setting should be concise and clear, and should address the *unusual*, not the routine, aspects of care. They should also be readily accessible for directing nursing care on a day-to-day basis and for directing documentation of key aspects of care.

Many hospitals are going through "growing pains" in developing their methods and forms for care planning. Some are struggling with lengthy documentation requirements, while others are moving toward more succinct computerized care planning systems. Some are placing their care plans on the chart, while others are keeping them at the bedside. Many hospitals are moving away from using just one page to address *all* nursing diagnoses to using

---

* Collaborative problems may also be addressed if they are unusual or complex, and are not covered by medical orders or hospital standards.

separate sheets for each diagnosis (see next page). This is because the column format that lists assessment, diagnosis, planning, and implementation across the top of the page can restrict nurses in how they write a plan of care. Nurses should continue to voice their needs during these times of change: *care plans are intended to assist staff nurses to deliver effective and efficient care*. If they do not (*e.g.*, if they are too cumbersome or not readily accessible), they should be reevaluated. Those who are involved in developing care planning systems should focus on how care plans are used, and choose methods that are realistic and acceptable to the nursing staff.

Page 132 offers guidelines for documenting care plans. To help you to avoid making errors, Display 4-3 gives examples of common errors on nursing care plans.

Pages 126–131 show several sample care plans. Page 126 is organized according to Orem's theory of self-care, and page 128 according to Gordon's Functional Health Patterns. Page 130 offers an example of a standardized care plan format for the nursing diagnosis of *Stress Incontinence*. This format has been designed to guide the nurse in writing a comprehensive, individualized plan of care for that specific diagnosis, and to save time-consuming repetitious documentation by having a "fill-in-the-blank" system. It has also been designed for easy transferral to a computerized system of care planning.

(*Text continues on page 132*)

Display 4-3. *Common Errors on Nursing Care Plans*

☐ Listing a problem that is already covered by hospital policy, standards, or physicians' orders.
Example: Potential for Infection related to central venous line. (This problem is not unusual, and should be covered by hospital policies and physicians' orders.)

☐ Calling a collaborative problem a nursing diagnosis.
Example: Altered Patterns of Urinary Elimination related to Foley catheter. (Foley catheters are collaborative problems.)

☐ Writing a nursing order that is already covered by a physician's order.
Example: Give pain medication as needed. (It would be better to write something that complements the physician's order, such as "document effectiveness of pain medication," or "give medication for pain exactly on time.")

☐ Omitting documentation orders.
Example: Writing "auscultate lung sounds" instead of "document lung sounds once a shift."

NURSING CARE PLAN

Date	Nursing Diagnosis	Expected Outcomes	Target Date	Resol Date

	Ineffective Breathing Pattern
	
	related to _neuro-muscular imp-airment_
	
	as evidenced by _C-6 Spinal cord injury, poor chest expansion_
	
	Common Etiologies
	
	Neuromuscular
	  Impairment
	Pain
	Musculoskeletal
	  Impairment
	Inflammatory Process
	Anxiety
	Decreased Lung
	  Expansion
	Decreased Energy or
	  Fatigue
	Infection
	Tracheo-Bronchial
	  Obstruction
	Structural Damage
		1. Achieve optimal lung expansion with adequate ventilation.
		
		X Identify causative factors and relate adaptive ways of coping with them.
		
		3. Remain free of signs and symptoms of hypoxia.
		
		4. Relate relief of symptoms and comfort in breathing
		
		5. Demonstrates effective breathing techniques and use of assistive devices.
			LTG
			
			Strength. Knows this well
			
			LTG
			
			LTG
			
			LTG	

Figure 4-2. Sample page from a nursing care plan that uses a separate page for each nursing diagnosis. (Adapted with permission of Bryn Mawr Hospital, Bryn Mawr, PA)

Nursing Interventions	Date IMP/DC	Nursing Orders	Date IMP/DC
1. Assess causative or contributing factors.	5/10	① Auscultate lungs q 4⁰ + prn + chart q 8⁰	
2. Reduce or eliminate causative or contributing factors, if possible.	5/10		
3. Assist patient in use of respiratory devices and techniques.	5/10	② Monitor use of incentive spirometer (he tries to skip when he's tired).	
4. Provide for adequate rest periods between treatments.	5/10		
5. Promote comfort.	5/10	③ Reinforce need for practicing "quad cough"!	
6. Provide emotional support.	5/10	④ Encourage family to assist him to ↑ mobility + in turning from side to side.	
7. Maintain adequate ventilation.	5/10		
8. Assess for signs and symptoms of hypoxia.	5/10		
9. Initiate health teaching and referrals as indicated.	5/10	⑤ Document vital capacity and NIF q 8⁰ on flow sheet. RA.	

Health Focus: Life Cycle
Long-Term Goal: Mrs. J. will react with other residents and become more involved in activities by 12/5/85.

Assessment Data	Nursing Diagnosis/ Collaborative Problem
10/15 *Therapeutic self-care demand:* Universal/Balance between activity & rest. *Related signs and symptoms:* Sleeps in a chair much of the day. States she's bored. Affect is flat. *Strengths:* Alert, oriented, pleasant, clear. Communicates well. Enjoys company, TV, gardening, music. Knowledgeable. *Limitations:* Has chronic low back pain. Confined to wheel chair. *Self-care deficit (knowledge, attitude, skills):* Lack of environmental stimuli and activity	Diversional Activity Deficit R/T inability to perform ADL as manifested by statements of "there's nothing I can do here."
10/15 *Therapeutic self-care demand:* Health deviation: back pain. *Related signs and symptoms:* c/o constant low back pain & asking for "pain killers." States she wishes she could control pain. *Strengths:* Willing to learn & do anything to reduce pain so she can walk independently again. Aware of effects of immobility. *Limitations:* Anxious, advanced age, Hx of partial compression fx L1, prosthesis r. hip, little family support. *Self-care deficit: (knowledge, attitude, skills):* Lacks knowledge of pain management techniques.	Impaired Physical Mobility R/T pain

Figure 4-3. *Sample care plan organized according to Orem's self-care theory. (Adapted from Holy Family College Nursing Department, Philadelphia, PA)*

Outcome	Nursing System/ Nursing Orders	Progress/Evaluation

10/15
1. Will report activities she en-
   joys doing by 10/16/85.
2. Will perform at least 2 activ-
   ities a day by 10/20/85.
3. Will report less boredom by
   10/20.
4. Will sleep 8 hrs. at night by
   10/20.
	Nursing System: Partially
	compensatory
	Nursing Orders: 10/15
	1. Assess activity level.
	2. Suggest some activities to do
	   (likes playing Bingo, cards, &
	   watching out window).
	3. Encourage her to make sug-
	   gestions and express ideas.
	4. Maintain lighted, cheerful en-
	   vironment.
	5. Make daily routine as normal
	   as possible.
	            M. Malloon, RN
		States she likes Bingo, cards,
		synagog, sitting by win-
		dow. MM
		10/20
		Will attend Bingo and goes to
		synagog if encouraged. MM
		Attended exercise class, but
		needs constant encour-
		agement. MM
		States she enjoys the activi-
		ties, but she does not seem
		to remember much about
		them.
		Sleeping 6–8 hours most
		nights. MM

1. Will report lessening of pain
   using a ten-point scale by
   10/25.
2. Will discuss techniques for ↓
   pain experience by 10/25.
3. Will be less dependent on
   medications by 10/25.
4. Will verbalize importance of
   ambulating by 10/18.
5. Will attempt to take small
   steps with walker by 10/25.
	Nursing System: Partially
	compensatory
	Nursing Orders: 10/15
	1. Assess low back pain q shift
	   and report abnormalities
	   (e.g., edema, bruising, red-
	   ness).
	2. Massage q 4 hrs.
	3. Perform ROM.
	4. Encourage her to wear brace
	   OOB.
	5. Medicate prn. Coach her in
	   relaxation techniques.
	6. Assist her to walk with walker
	   t.i.d. M. Malloon, RN
		10/25
		Rates pain at #2 level (less).
		                 MM
		Relates that back rubs &
		massages reduce pain. MM
		Still needs medication q 4 hr.
		                 MM
		10/18
		Verbalizes that she should try
		to walk more to keep up
		strength. MM
		10/25
		Can walk from bed to bath-
		room with walker. MM

Assessment Data	Nursing Diagnosis/ Collaborative Problem
10/20 *Health management/Health perception:* Nonsmoker. Goes to aerobic 3 × wk when well. States being ill and dependent on others is very difficult on her. *Nutrition/metabolic pattern:* 20 lb overweight. Has had no appetite since illness started 10 days ago. Has had fever of 101 much of the time. Skin intact—no rashes. *Elimination pattern:* BM q other day usually. Now has diarrhea 10–15×/day. Has external hemorrhoids. Urine dark and concentrated. *Activity/exercise pattern:* Has not been out of house for past 10 days. Feels she is too weak to go out. *Cognitive perception pattern:* College graduate. Alert and appropriate in communication.	10/20 1. Fluid Volume Deficit R/T Fever, diarrhea, and loss of appetite as manifested by dark concentrated urine. 2. Diarrhea R/T unknown etiology.
10/20 *Sleep/rest pattern:* Sleeps much of the time, but disturbed by having to get up to BR for diarrhea *Self-perception/self-concept pattern:* States she's an independent individual. *Role/relationship pattern:* Married. Has one child. Worried because she says husband is "not good" with daughter. *Sexual/reproductive pattern:* Married. Other data collection deferred. *Coping/stress pattern:* States she's a "doer"—likes to be active doing things when she is depressed. *Value/belief pattern:* Catholic. Attends Mass most Sundays.	10/20 3. Possible Altered Family Processes R/T illness of mother 4. Potential Impaired Skin Integrity (rectal area) R/T diarrhea & hemorrhoids.

Figure 4-4. *Sample care plan organized according to Gordon's functional health patterns.*

Outcome	Nursing Orders	Evaluation
Will maintain hydration by drinking at least 2000 ml per day every day.	10/20 1. Keep ginger ale with juice at bedside. 2. Force fluids (clear liq) to: 1000 ml (7–3) 750 ml (3–11) 250 ml (7–11) 3. Assess fluid intake every 2 hours while awake. 4. Both nurse & pt should keep a record of I/O. 5. Monitor electrolyte studies. J. Martin RN	10/22 Fluid intake only 1500 ml last 2 days. Discussed her need to push more. JM Electrolytes WNL JM Urine output 700 cc and concentrated. JM Keeping own I/O record. JM
Will develop normal bowel movements by controlling diarrhea through medication and diet by 10/22.	10/20 1. Maintain clear liquid diet. 2. Assess BMs q 3° while awake and give Lomotil prn. J. Martin RN	10/22 Diarrhea ↓ to 4 × day. Clear liquids maintained. Taking Lomotil q.i.d. JM
She and her husband will discuss how family will cope with illness by 10/22.	10/20 Spend time discussing with husband and wife together and separately to determine how the family is adapting to illness and to identify potential problems. J. Martin RN	10/22 Husband has not been to visit for longer than 10 minutes, and I have missed him both times. Told her to ask him to call me when he can. JM
Rectal area will remain clean and without signs of irritation.	Encourage warm sitz baths qid especially p̄ BMs J. Martin RN	10/22 Taking sitz bath. Rectal area clean–not red. JM

Patient Name: _____	The Bryn Mawr Hospital
Room Number: _____	Nursing Service Department
	NURSING CARE PLAN

Date/ Ident	Nursing Diagnosis	Expected Outcomes	Target Date	Resol Date
	Stress Incontinence related to: (*Specify*) _____ _____ _____ as evidenced by: (*Choose from below*). _____ _____ _____ <u>Common Etiologies</u> Weak Pelvic Muscles and Structural Supports Obesity Pregnancy Incompetent Bladder Outlet Overdistention Between Voidings Decreased Bladder Capacity <u>Identify Initials</u> ____ _____ ____ _____ ____ _____ ____ _____ ____ _____ ____ _____	(*Circle appropriate outcomes below*) 1. Relate under-standing of causa-tive and contri-buting factors. 2. Verbalize feelings of frustration and/or embarrassment. 3. Receive adequate information regard-ing interventions and hygienic aids. 4. Maintain optimal skin integrity.		

Figure 4-5. *Example of care plan form that uses a "fill in the blank" system. (Adapted with permission of Bryn Mawr Hospital, Bryn Mawr, PA)*

Nursing Interventions	Date IMP/DC	Nursing Orders	Date IMP/DC
1. Assess causative or contributing factors.		*(List individualized interventions below. Use the interventions listed to the left as a guide.)*	
2. Reduce or eliminate causative or contributing factors, if possible.			
3. Assist patient in use of respiratory devices and techniques.			
4. Provide for adequate rest periods between treatments.			
5. Promote comfort.			
6. Provide emotional support.			
7. Maintain adequate ventilation.			
8. Assess for signs and symptoms of hypoxia.			
9. Initiate health teaching and referrals as indicated.			

     Documenting Care Plans

☐ Be sure that diagnoses, expected outcomes, nursing orders, and evaluation are addressed on each care plan.

☐ List only those nursing diagnoses and collaborative problems that vary from routine or standard care.

☐ Be brief, but be clear:

Use accepted abbreviations (*e.g.*, NPO, OOB).

Use key words rather than full sentences.

Refer nurses to procedure manuals for routine and standard care procedures.

☐ List long- and short-term goals (when appropriate), and set target dates for goal achievement.

☐ Indicate dates when goals are set and met.

Problem-Oriented Medical Records (POMR)

Some institutions use Problem-Oriented Medical Records (POMR) to document the plan of care. POMR is a method of charting the patient's plan of care whereby all members of the healthcare team document patient problems in the same place on the chart (called the problem list). For example, if you were to look at the problem list for a particular patient, you may find problems that have been identified by physicians, nurses, dietitians, and physical therapists. The problems are listed in order of when they were identified, not necessarily in order of priority. Table 4-4 shows a sample problem list.

Table 4-4. Problem List

Date of Diagnosis	Problem	Date Resolved
1/5	1. Cerebrovascular accident (identified by physician)	
	2. Potential Impaired Skin Integrity related to immobility (identified by nursing)	
	3. Unsteady gait (identified by physical therapist)	
1/7	4. Altered Self-Concept related to loss of ability to move right side (identified by nursing)	
1/8	5. Urinary tract infection (identified by physician)	1/13

Institutions that use POMR feel that listing all the problems in one place will increase communication among the members of the healthcare team; each member working with the patient will be aware of *all* of the problems for that particular patient.

SOAP Charting.   The use of POMR requires that all members of the healthcare team use a method of charting called SOAP charting. SOAP charting includes documentation of the following information on the patient's chart:

S = Subjective data (what the patient tells you about his problem)

O = Objective data (what is observed about the patient's problem)

A = Assessment/analysis (problem statement)

P = Plan (goals and interventions)

Display 4-4 shows an example of SOAP charting.

SOAPIE Charting.   SOAPIE charting, an expanded form of SOAP charting, is closer to the nursing process in format because it includes the steps of implementation and evaluation.

S = Subjective data

O = Objective data

A = Assessment

P = Plan

I = Interventions (implementation)

E = Evaluation

At present, SOAP charting is often used for the initial assessment of the patient, and SOAPIE charting is used after implementation of the care has progressed to the point at which evaluation is appropriate.

Display 4-4.   SOAP Charting

S: "I feel so helpless because I can't move since I had my stroke."

O: Unable to move right side of body
Slouched in bed in half sitting position
Has reddened area about 5 cm around coccyx

A: Potential Impaired Skin Integrity related to immobility

P: Prevent skin breakdown:

Reposition side to side every 2 hours when in bed

Assist out of bed three times a day for 1/2 hour

Acquire sheepskin for coccyx area

Massage coccyx with lotion q.i.d. and p.r.n.

Key Points Planning

1. The third step of the nursing process, planning, involves the following activities:

    Setting priorities

    Establishing client goals/expected outcomes

    Determining nursing actions

    Documenting the nursing care plan

2. When you establish a plan of nursing care, you must apply standards that are set by the law, the ANA, and the institution where you are working.

3. Setting priorities during the *initial planning stage* includes the following:

    ☐ Determining the problems that need immediate attention and taking immediate action

    ☐ Determining the nursing diagnoses that will be addressed on the nursing care plan (those that are unusual or complex)

    ☐ Determining the collaborative problems that require physician's orders for diagnosis, monitoring, or treatment

4. Setting priorities requires insight into the entire picture and an awareness of how all of the problems are affecting the individuals involved.

5. Setting *realistic goals* is an important activity of planning for the following reasons:

    ☐ They are the "measuring sticks" of the plan of care.

    ☐ They direct your interventions.

    ☐ They are motivating factors.

6. *Client-centered goals* focus upon the desired end result of the plan of care: that the client benefits from nursing care.

7. Writing expected outcomes involves writing goals in three domains:

    Cognitive Domain: Outcomes that are associated with changes in knowledge or intellectual abilities

    Affective Domain: Outcomes that are associated with changes in attitudes, feelings, or values

    Psychomotor Domain: Outcomes that deal with developing motor skills

8. Verbs used in writing expected outcomes/goals should be measurable verbs that describe the exact behavior that you expect to *see* or *hear*.

9. Nursing interventions include assessing, doing, counseling, referring, and teaching.

10. To be sure of being comprehensive when writing nursing orders, you should consider what you want nurses to assess, to do, to teach, and to document.

11. Nursing orders should give clear instructions about what nursing actions should be implemented for each specific problem, including the following components:

    Date: The date the order was written

    Verb: The action that is to be performed

    Subject: Who is going to perform the action

    Descriptive Phrase: How, when, where, how often, how long, how much

    Signature of the Nurse: Whoever wrote it should sign it

12. Standard care plans should be used *only as a guide* with thoughtful analysis on your part as a nurse. (See Guidelines: Individualizing Standard Care Plans.)

13. Nursing care plans focus upon the plan of care for *nursing diagnoses*, and serve three major purposes: to direct nursing interventions, to direct nursing documentation, and to provide a tool for evaluation.

14. Methods of documenting care plans vary from institution to institution because they must meet the unique needs of the nurses and patients in that particular institution. However, they should all provide for documentation of nursing diagnoses, expected outcomes, nursing interventions, and evaluation.

Bibliography

American Nurses' Association (1973) *Standards of Nursing Practice.* Kansas City, MO.

Beck, J. (1980) Standards as a guide for nursing care plans. *Oncol. Nurs. Forum* 7(4):28–30.

Carpenito, L. (1987) *Handbook of Nursing Diagnosis.* 2nd ed. Philadelphia: JB Lippincott.

Carpenito, L. (1987) *Nursing Diagnosis: Application to Clinical Practice.* 2nd ed. Philadelphia: JB Lippincott.

Gordon, M. (1982) *Nursing Diagnosis: Process and Application.* New York: McGraw-Hill.

Griffith, J. and Christensen, P. (1982) *Nursing Process: Application of Theories, Frameworks and Models.* St. Louis: CV Mosby.

Maslow, A. (1970) *Motivation in Personality.* New York: Harper & Row.

Mathewman, J. (1987) Combining careplan and kardex. *Am. J. Nurs.* (6)87:852–854.

Orem, D. (1980) *Nursing: Concepts of Practice.* 2nd ed. New York: McGraw-Hill.

Uhrich, S., Canale, S., and Wendell, S. (1986) *Nursing Care Planning Guides: A Nursing Process Approach.* Philadelphia: WB Saunders.

Vogelberger, M. (1986) A new approach to the care-plan problem. *J. Nurs. Staff Dev.* 2(3):120–125.

☑ Continuing Data Collection
☑ Setting Daily Priorities
☑ Performing Nursing Interventions
☑ Documenting Nursing Care (Charting)
☑ Giving Verbal Nursing Reports
☑ Maintaining a Current Care Plan

5
Implementation

Standard V: *Nursing actions provide for client/patient participation in health promotion, maintenance, and restoration.*

Standard VI: *Nursing actions assist the client/patient to maximize his health capabilities.**

*Abstracted from Standards of Nursing Practice. Copyright American Nurses' Association, 1973

Glossary

Charting A method of documenting factual, concise, descriptive data to communicate patient assessments and nursing interventions performed by and for the patient. (This documentation often provides the most recent communication of the patient's status, and is used as a way of measuring the success of nursing care.)

Putting the Plan Into Action

You have identified problems and strengths, and you have determined a goal-oriented, individualized plan of action; now you are ready for implementation. Let's take a look at the process of putting the plan into action. This chapter will first discuss the relationship between planning and implementation, then focus upon the "how-to's" of the following activities of the implementation phase:

☐ Continuing data collection and assessment

☐ Setting daily priorities

☐ Performing nursing interventions

☐ Documentation nursing care (charting)

☐ Giving verbal nursing reports

☐ Maintaining a current care plan

Relationship of Planning to Implementation

Planning and implementation are closely related: during planning you determine nursing orders to direct interventions, and during implementation you actually perform the interventions. This close relationship can be confusing for students. When writing care plans to describe patient care, students often write the same thing under planning and implementation. For example, a student may write under planning, "Get the patient out of bed 3 times today," and then under implementation, "Got the patient out of bed 3 times today." The key point to remember is that in planning you write orders for interventions, while in implementation you follow the orders, but you *also assess the patient before, during, and after the interventions are performed.* (In the above example, the student forgot to describe, under implementation, assessments of the patient's condition before getting out of bed, while he was out of bed, and after he got out of bed.)

Planning gives direction to implementation but prescribed interventions are performed only when appropriate, *as indicated by ongoing data collection.*

Continuing Data Collection

Ongoing data collection provides the necessary information to make decisions about whether the prescribed plan of care is appropriate. Depending on your assessment of a situation, you must be ready to change actions as necessary;

interventions that may have been appropriate yesterday may be useless, or even harmful, today.

Ongoing data collection may also provide *key information* about the appropriateness of a patient's nursing diagnoses. Since many institutions require documentation of nursing diagnoses within the first 24 hours of admission, it will not be unusual for you to change a diagnosis or add or delete a diagnosis, based upon additional patient information.

The time that you spend performing specific or routine nursing activities can be a valuable time for further data collection. For example, the simple procedure of giving a bedbath or back rub can yield important data about the physical and mental status of your patient. During these procedures, you can gain information about your patient's physical status by making observations such as the condition of his skin and his ability to move; and you can gain information about his mental status by using therapeutic communication techniques to encourage him to verbalize feelings or concerns. Note the following example:

> During the nursing report, the evening nurse had been told that Mrs. Sowers seemed to be a somewhat "difficult" patient. She had been admitted for studies of her gastrointestinal tract, but was otherwise in good general health. Mrs. Sowers spent the entire day in bed, and the nursing staff had been concerned because they had decided that she should be ambulating to maintain her strength. However, Mrs. Sowers had verbalized that she was too tired to walk much and that she wanted to rest in bed. The nurses had described her as being a somewhat dependent person who was very quiet and introverted. That evening, the nurse went in to give Mrs. Sowers a back rub and to help her get settled for bed. While giving the back rub, the nurse mentioned to Mrs. Sowers that she seemed very tired all the time. She then asked if there was something that was causing her to feel this way. Mrs. Sowers responded by explaining that she had not slept well in weeks because she had just found out her daughter had breast cancer and she was very frightened that she might die. This was important information that had never been offered before. The nurse was then able to talk with Mrs. Sowers about her fears and concerns and to offer a positive outlook by explaining that breast cancer, when detected early, has a good prognosis. By ten o'clock that night, Mrs. Sowers was not only up ambulating, but also helping her roommate by offering her sips of juice, and so forth.

The above situation exemplifies the importance of ongoing data collection during the performance of routine interventions.

Setting Daily Priorites

The ability to set daily priorities is the key to implementing a plan of care. Even the best-laid plan cannot predict what will happen *on a day-to-day basis*. You will have to learn to assess situations on a day-to-day (even moment-to-moment) basis, and to be flexible. Often you will find yourself "juggling the schedule" to facilitate optimum treatment of several different problems during the course of the day. Page 92 (Chap. 4) offers basic principles for setting priorities during the *initial* planning stage, which can also be applied to setting priorities on a day-to-day basis. If you are a student, it will be worthwhile to take a moment to review these principles so that you can apply them as you read this section.

Your ability to set priorities will depend upon your nursing knowledge and expertise, and your knowledge of routines at the facility where you work. However, let's take a look at some suggested steps that can be used *as a guide* when determining priorities on a daily basis.

Suggested Steps for Setting Daily Priorities

Step #1. Before you determine priorities, study medical and nursing records (including the care plan), pay close attention to change-of-shift reports, *and assess the patient yourself.*

Rationale: How you prioritize problems will be influenced by change-of-shift reports and assessment of medical and nursing records. However, it is important that you take the time to verify this information by *direct patient assessment* to be sure that the status of problems has not changed.

Step #2. Take time to briefly assess *critical problems* before you perform a more in-depth assessment of all the problems.

Rationale: Verification of critical data (*e.g.*, rates of IV infusion, status of invasive lines, operation of equipment, physical status of critical patients) should be done immediately after (or before or during) the change-of-shift report. This prevents misunderstandings and helps both the oncoming nurse and the offgoing nurse to settle problems while both are available to each other for clarification.

Step #3. Depending upon your assessment, determine any problems that need to be resolved immediately, and take appropriate action (*e.g.*, report to head nurse, instructor, or physician, and implement independent interventions, as appropriate).

Rationale: Setting the wheels in motion to correct severe problems takes priority over taking time to analyze *all* the patient's problems.

Step #4. List the problems (nursing diagnoses and collaborative problems) and ask the following questions:

☐ Are there any problems that I must resolve today (and what happens if I wait till later)?

☐ What are the problems that I must monitor today (and what could happen if I do not)?

☐ What are the key problems that I must resolve, reduce, or control today to achieve the overall goals of care?

☐ Of three problems, which two can I realistically work on today? (If you have more problems, then, of course, you would work on more.)

Rationale: Answering the above questions will help you to determine what *must* be done today.

Step #5.   Having listed your problems for today, determine the tasks that must be done to work toward their resolution. List these tasks and routine tasks, such as baths, meals, *etc.*

Rationale: Often you will be performing tasks to work on several of the problems during the course of the day, but not necessarily resolving any one of the problems completely. For example, you may be giving a routine bedbath to promote hygiene, and at the same time using therapeutic communication to discuss problems with coping.

Step #6.   Together with the patient, study your list of tasks to determine the things that the patient and family can do on their own, and the things that require your assistance.

Rationale: The patient and family should be included in determining when things will get done, and they should be encouraged to be as independent as possible. Sometimes, patients need to be given permission to be independent.

Step #7.   Make a detailed personal worksheet for getting things done for the day, and *refer to it frequently.* Be sure to consider the daily routine of the unit (*e.g.,* when meals are served).

Rationale: You are likely to experience many distractions during the course of the day, and you should not rely on memory. While the daily routine of the unit should not *dictate* your activities, it will be vital to consider when setting the schedule.

Performing Nursing Interventions

Performing nursing interventions includes the following:

☐ Directly performing an activity for a client

☐ Assisting the client to perform an activity himself

☐ Supervising the client (or family) while he performs an activity himself

☐ Teaching the client (or family) about his healthcare

☐ Counseling the client (or family) in making choices about seeking and utilizing appropriate healthcare resources

☐ Monitoring (assessing) the client for potential complications/problems

Chapter 4 (Planning) discusses how to determine specific nursing interventions for specific problems. This section will discuss how interventions, in general, should be implemented.

The tasks involved in performing nursing interventions can vary from simple to complex. However, there are some activities that are common to almost all interventions. The acronym "cwipat" is suggested to help you to remember the common tasks that you should perform with every nursing intervention. "Cwipat" stands for the following:

C = Check the orders and equipment.

W = Wash your hands.

I = Identify the patient.

P = Provide for safety and privacy.

A = Assess the problem.

T = *Tell* the person or *Teach* the person about what you are going to do.

Making sure that you do all the steps suggested by the word "cwipat" before you perform a nursing intervention helps to organize the nursing procedure and reduce the possibility of error.

The following guidelines are suggested to help beginners when implementing (performing) nursing interventions.

☐ *Guidelines*   *Performing Nursing Interventions*

☐ Never perform a nursing intervention until you know the reason (rationale) for performing the activity, the expected effect of the activity, the possible side effects of the activity, and the possible adverse effects of the activity.

☐ Before you implement a nursing action, you must reassess your patient to determine the status of the problem and whether the interventions previously identified are still appropriate (*i.e.*, perform a focus assessment).

☐ Performing nursing interventions cannot be a rote or mechanical activity. You must continually assess the response of the patient to your nursing interventions and be ready to change interventions that are not working.

☐ When you perform nursing interventions, you should include the patient and his family. Always explain why you are performing the intervention.

☐ Nursing interventions should be accomplished in a safe and therapeutic environment. Plan ahead to be sure the environment is appropriate for whatever activity is going to be performed.

☐ Be sure that you are aware of institutional protocols and procedures, which often vary from institution to institution.

Documenting Nursing Care (Charting)

Charting, or documentation of nursing care, is a legal requirement of all healthcare systems. There are no ifs, ands, or buts—you must learn to chart, and you must learn to chart well. The nursing notes that you will be writing will become a part of the client's permanent legal record, a record that may later be introduced as evidence in a court of law. These notes will be the most current written communication of what has happened to the patient during the course of the day. Poor, illegible, or incomplete charting may impede nursing care because it will be more difficult to recognize significant changes in health status without the clear documentation of client activities and behaviors. Good, factually descriptive nursing notes will enhance patient care because they will communicate the pertinent aspects of the client's healthcare and help others to assess patterns of client responses.

You will notice that forms used for charting nurses' notes will vary because each healthcare facility needs to have a method of documentation that *meets its particular requirements*. Even though these forms may differ in appearance, they must all provide for documentation of observations and occurrences according to exact time and sequence of events. Often this documentation will provide the only answers to questions that may arise about a client's healthcare. Nurses' notes may offer the only proof that medical and nursing treatments have indeed been carried out. This information may later be necessary for insurance purposes and for evaluation of nursing care.

Just as with nursing assessments, there are two types of nurses' notes. One is the comprehensive notes that are written at the time of the initial contact with a client, and the other is the problem-focused notes that are written about specific problems. Chapter 2 offers examples of forms for documenting an initial comprehensive data base assessment (see pages 17–27). Figure 5-1 shows an example of a problem-focused nursing note that has been written for

Date and Time	Problems/Diagnoses	Nursing Assessments and Comments
5/8/90 8 AM	#1 Potential Ineffective Airway Clearance related to thick secretions #2 Potential Fluid Volume Deficit related to poor fluid intake	Coughing up thick white mucus—he does this well, but needs to be reminded to work at it. Lungs have a few scattered rhonchi at both bases. Fluids encouraged—he does drink juices well—apple juice on ice kept at bedside. ————————————————H. Laird RN
10:30 AM		OOB to chair for ½ hour. States he feels very fatigued, but he is steady on his feet.
10:45 AM		Voided lge amount clear yellow urine. Allowed to rest before pulmonary function test. ——— ————————————————H. Laird RN
11:30 AM		To special studies via wheelchair for pulmonary function. ——————————H. Laird RN
12:30 PM		Returned via wheelchair. Assisted back to bed. Ate all of his lunch—said it was the first time he's been hungry. ——————H. Laird RN

Figure 5-1. *Example of Problem-Focused Nurses' Notes.*

a patient with the nursing diagnosis of *Potential Ineffective Airway Clearance related to thick secretions.*

You will notice quite a difference in the amount of information that is charted with each type of nurses' notes. Patients with more acute and complex problems will require more frequent, in-depth, and comprehensive nursing notes. Patients with less severe problems are more likely to require problem-focused nursing notes that are shorter and less comprehensive.

In an effort to make daily charting more efficient, many hospitals are working to change their forms and requirements. As you move from one healthcare facility to another, you will have to become familiar with both the charting forms and the responsibilities for charting, as set forth in standards, policy, and procedure manuals of each institution. Although the forms, standards, policies, and procedure manuals may differ from one place to another, the basic content of nursing notes is similar. The following guidelines are suggested to help beginners to learn how to chart efficiently and effectively.

☐ *Guidelines*   *Charting Nurses' Notes*

☐ Use ink and be legible. Print if your handwriting is not clear.

☐ Write your notes as soon as possible after giving nursing care so that your recall will be most accurate.

☐ Be precise. Write down exactly how, when, and where the events and activities occurred.

EXAMPLE

4/29/90 9:10 A.M.—Ambulated for 15 min. to the end of the hall and back with wife's assistance. Gait is steady, and he says he is "feeling stronger."

☐ Always sign your first initial, last name, and credentials after each entry that you complete (*e.g.,* F. Nightingale, R.N.).

☐ Never leave a blank line; draw a line through unused spaces before and after your signature. (Note the example on the next page.)

☐ Include the following in your nurses' notes:

Assessment: What you see, hear, smell, or observe about the current physical and emotional status of the client

Intervention: The activities performed by the client, yourself, family, or other members of the healthcare team

Evaluation: The response of the client to activities and interventions performed

☐ Be concise, yet descriptive. You do not have to write complete sentences, but use adjectives and accepted abbreviations to give a good picture of activities and observations.

☐ Be specific. Avoid using vague terms.

Date Time	Vital Signs				Fluids		Nursing Notes
	Temp	Pulse	Resp.	B/P	Intake	Output	
4/20/86 7:30AM	98⁴	92	20		78	200	Assisted to B.R. Refused bkfst. c/o nausea. S. Jones R.N.————
8:30AM		88	20				A.M. care given Abd. dsg. dry. S. Jones R.N.————
9:45AM		84	16				Dr. Witt here. S. Jones R.N.————
10:50AM	98⁴	110	20				c/o shooting, sharp incisional pain. Quarter size pink drainage noted on abd. dsg. Requests pain med.——— S. Jones R.N.————

EXAMPLE:

Wrong: Noted moderate amount of drainage on abdominal dressing.

Right: Abdominal dressing has an area of light pink drainage about 6 inches in diameter.

☐ Be complete. Remember the adage, "If it wasn't charted, it wasn't done." If you fail to chart medications or significant actions delivered *or* withheld, it may result in an adverse reaction, overdose, or perhaps even death.

☐ Use examples and the client's own words to clarify your description of what you observe or infer.

EXAMPLE:

Wrong: "Appears uncomfortable."

Right: "Doesn't seem to get good pain relief—he states that he is 'OK' but he moves stiffly and constantly holds his side."

☐ Always document variations from the norm (*e.g.*, abnormalities in respiration, circulation, mental status, or behavior).

☐ Always document the status of invasive lines/treatment modalities (*e.g.*, oxygen therapy, traction, Foley catheters, nasogastric tubes, intravenous lines).

☐ Do not use the word "patient." Since it is the patient's chart, it is assumed.

Display 5-1 lists the criteria that good charting systems should have.

Display 5-1. Criteria for Good Charting Systems

Good charting systems should

- Be tailor-made to the types of problems frequently demonstrated by the patient population of the facility, to direct nurses to chart the key aspects of patient care.
- Discourage double documentation (charting the same thing in two different places) and irrelevant charting.
- Be designed so that crucial patient data (*e.g.,* focus assessments and interventions for specific problems) are easily retrievable, and so that the method of charting can save the nurse's time without reducing the quality of charting (*e.g.,* flow sheets).

Recommended reading: Burke, L. and Murphy, J. (1988) *Charting by Exception.* New York: John Wiley & Sons.

☐ *Practice Session*   *Charting Nurses' Notes*
(*Suggested Answers on page 178*)

Study the two case situations listed below. Then, using the forms provided on pages 148 and 149 (or using your own form), write the nursing notes that you would record given the data presented for each situation.

Case A

Today you are Mr. Johns's nurse. He is a smoker and was admitted 2 days ago with chronic lung disease. He has the nursing diagnosis of *Potential Ineffective Airway Clearance related to thick mucus secretions.* When you enter his room at 8:30 A.M., he is sitting in a chair and seems to be wheezing more than usual. You note that he is using accessory muscles of the chest to help him breathe. His breakfast tray is sitting in front of him untouched. When you tell him that he seems to be having more trouble breathing, he replies, "Nope, I'm okay—I'm just a little tired, that's all." He refuses to eat because he says he is not hungry.

Ten minutes later, you enter the room to take his vital signs. His temperature is 97°F. His pulse is 130 and regular. His blood pressure is 170/94. His respiratory status is essentially unchanged with a rate of 32, but his behavior has changed. He is now more restless and is not sure that he is still in the hospital. You assist him into bed, put up the side rails, raise the head of the bed, and begin oxygen at 2 liters/min via nasal cannula. He still appears to be in respiratory distress. You notify the physician about these changes.

At 9:00 A.M., the physician examines the patient and orders arterial blood gases to be drawn by the lab and breathing treatments to begin immediately.

At 9:10 A.M., the lab draws blood gases and asks you to maintain pressure on the arterial puncture site for 5 minutes. You do this, and note that the site has no bleeding after 5 minutes.

At 9:15 A.M., the respiratory therapist comes in and administers the breathing treatment. Mr. Johns then coughs up a large amount of thick white mucus.

At 9:35 A.M., you reassess Mr. Johns and find that his lungs are more clear. He no longer seems confused, and he agrees to take a few sips of water.

At 10:00 A.M., Mr. Johns is much improved and asks to get out of bed. You discontinue his oxygen and assist him to a chair. His pulse is 110, and respirations are 28.

Case B

Tonight you are Mrs. Fox's nurse. Mrs. Fox is a newly diagnosed diabetic who has the nursing diagnosis of *Knowledge Deficit: Self-administration of Insulin.*

You have taught Mrs. Fox how to give her own insulin injection, and she has given herself her first injection that morning without problems. You walk into the room at 5:00 P.M. to supervise her in giving herself her pre-dinner insulin. Mrs. Fox follows the procedure for withdrawing the insulin, but contaminates the needle before she injects herself. You point this out to her, and she replies, "Well, it only barely touched the sheet when I put it down for a moment." You reinforce the importance of maintaining sterile technique.

She eats all her dinner. At 8:00 P.M., she states that she's "dying for a chocolate bar" and that she feels that the diabetic diet is going to be impossible to follow. You discuss the possibility of talking with the dietician about possible modifications in diet and point out that she is scheduled for a fruit snack at 9:00 P.M. You suggest that perhaps she could do something to get her mind off her desire for food. She decides to call her friend on the phone to chat.

At 9:00 P.M., you bring her fruit snack and a small glass of milk. She eats it all.

At 9:30 P.M., you spend a half-hour discussing how Mrs. Fox feels she is progressing with all the changes in her life. She is more optimistic and states, "You know, I'm beginning to feel as though I'll get through all this. I've almost got the injection bit down pat, and with a bit of help, maybe I'll get my diet straightened out too."

At 10:00 P.M., Mrs. Fox is quietly resting in bed.

Date and Time	Of Special Notation	Nursing Assessments and Comments

Date and Time	Of Special Notation	Nursing Assessments and Comments

Giving Verbal Nursing Reports

The verbal reports that you give concerning your patients can have a major influence on the overall healthcare that they receive. For example, look at the two verbal reports below. (Both examples are reports about the same patient.)

Verbal Nursing Report 1

"Mrs. J. has had her usual bad day. She is driving me crazy with her moaning and groaning about her back pain. I've given her everything I can, but she's still on the light all the time . . . and she even has her husband hopping around for every little request! The x-rays have been negative. This has been going on for 2 weeks! I wish they'd do something with her—I think she's just a crock, and this isn't a psychiatric unit. Her signs are stable, and intake and output okay. Good luck with her."

Verbal Nursing Report 2

"Mrs. J. seems to have had another bad day. She seems so uncomfortable. She states the pain medicine gives very little relief, if any. Her husband has been very supportive and tries to help her, but nothing seems to work. The x-rays have been negative. It must be really hard to be here for 2 weeks without getting any better or finding out what's wrong. I wish we could do more for her. Her signs are stable and she's had 700 ml intake today. She should be encouraged to drink more during the evening."

If you compare the two examples above, you will probably notice the negativism and subjectivity of Report 1. The nurse has begun to pass on the word that "this patient is a crock." If continued, the attitude of the whole nursing staff can become negative. On the other hand, the nurse in Report 2 passes on the report of "I wish we could do more for her," which is a much more positive message.

The importance of verbal nursing reports cannot be underestimated. A good, clear verbal report can enhance the quality of nursing care and promote greater continuity. A poor, highly subjective report can create errors and confusion. For these reasons, you must be sure that you can give an organized, clear, objective nursing report.

Because the change-of-shift report from a nurse who is going off duty to another nurse who is coming on duty is one of the most common forms of verbal nursing reports, let's take a look at some guidelines that you can follow when you give a change-of-shift report on your patients.

☐ *Guidelines*   *Giving a Change-of-Shift Report*

☐ Begin by giving basic background information, including the following: name, room number, age, attending and consulting physicians, date of admission, medical diagnoses, surgical procedures, and nursing diagnoses.

EXAMPLE:

"Mrs. Ballard, in room 214 by the window, is a 35-year-old patient of Dr. Smith, with a consultation to Dr. Jones. She was admitted on 5/25 with pneumonia. She had a tracheostomy on 5/26. Her nursing diagnoses are *Potential Ineffective Airway Clearance related to thick and copious secretions, Potential Impaired Skin Integrity related to bedrest,* and *Anxiety related to new situation of hospitalization* (has never been hospitalized before)."

☐ Give a general report on how the day went from the *patient's point of view,* rather than from your own point of view.

EXAMPLE:

Right: "Mr. Smith has not felt so well today."

Wrong: "I had a bad day with Mr. Smith."

☐ Don't be vague. Give specific observable data whenever possible.

EXAMPLES:

Right: "Mr. Smith has had an increase in his respiratory rate to 32/min. His heart rate is up to 122, and his temperature is 101."

Wrong: "Mr. Smith seems to be having respiratory difficulty."

Right: "I gave Mr. Smith 8 mg of morphine IM at 5:10 P.M. for incisional pain."

Wrong: "I gave Mr. Smith a pain med for his pain."

☐ When describing a problem, use the nursing process and describe assessment, diagnosis, planning, implementation, and evaluation in order to be sure that your report is organized.

EXAMPLE:

Right: "Mr. Smith complains of constipation. He hasn't had a bowel movement in 4 days. I gave him milk of magnesia and some prune juice this morning, but he still hasn't moved his bowels."

Wrong: "I gave Mr. Smith some milk of magnesia and some prune juice. He's constipated, and still has not moved his bowels. He hasn't gone in 4 days."

☐ If you make an inference, qualify your statement (*e.g.,* use a phrase such as "The patient seems to . . . ")

EXAMPLE:

Right: "Mr. Smith seems withdrawn to me."

Wrong: "Mr. Smith has been withdrawn today."

☐ Describe the presence of all invasive medical treatments (*e.g.*, intravenous lines, Foley catheters, nasogastric tubes).

☐ Stress abnormal findings (*e.g.*, rales in the lungs, abnormal vital signs).

☐ Stress variations from routine (*e.g.*, "This patient will *not* have a preop medication").

☐ Describe the nursing care that has been done, including the following:

Assessment of vital signs

Focus assessment of current nursing diagnosis/collaborative problems

Patient activities (*e.g.*, "Ambulated well . . . ")

Nursing interventions (*e.g.*, "Applied warm soaks . . . ")

Measurement of intake and output (if applicable)

Medical interventions (*e.g.*, "Inserted central venous line . . . ")

Diagnostic studies (*e.g.*, "Potassium was 3.8.")

☐ Describe the nursing care that has to be done, including the following:

Frequency of assessment of vital signs/specific assessment for potential complications (*e.g.*, "Observe for bleeding at catheter site").

Diet

Patient activities

Nursing interventions

Medical treatments

Diagnostic studies

Ongoing Evaluation/Maintaining a Current Care Plan

Even before you get to a formal evaluation period, you should be performing ongoing evaluation of both patient care and your own nursing activities on a daily basis. You should be asking yourself two questions:

1. How is each of my patients responding to my nursing care?

2. How are *my* days going?

As you perform nursing interventions, you should be evaluating the daily progress of each of your patients. If a patient is not progressing, you should begin to examine factors that are impeding progress (this will be discussed in Chapter 6, Evaluation). If a patient is progressing well, you may want to consider if perhaps your patient could be doing more or moving at a quicker pace. You may even note that some of the problems that you originally identified have changed or disappeared. It is important to make changes that are obviously necessary before you get to a formal evaluation phase. All these

> ### Display 5-2. Questions to Ask Yourself to Evaluate Your Work Day
>
> How has the day, in general, gone?
>
> Have I completed everything I should have?
>
> Have I been organized?
>
> Have I been able to set priorities well?
>
> What are some of the factors that have influenced how I have set priorities and organized my day?
>
> Am I identifying both nursing diagnoses and collaborative problems for my patients?
>
> How much time am I spending performing collaborative nursing interventions?
>
> How much time am I spending implementing independent nursing interventions?
>
> Could I be doing more?
>
> Am I trying to do too much?
>
> Are there changes I should make tomorrow?

changes should be documented on the nursing care plan so that all nurses who read the plan have a clear, up-to-date idea of the plan of care.

Revision of the care plan should include checking to be sure that the following information is up-to-date:

☐ Nursing diagnoses (and collaborative problems, if listed)

☐ Nursing orders (interventions)

☐ Goals/expected outcomes (with target dates for completion)

☐ Evaluation (reports on client progress)

(Modifying and revising the care plan will be further discussed in Chapter 6.)

In addition to evaluating patient progress, it is a good idea to take some time at the end of your day to determine if you, yourself, are having satisfactory days. Ask yourself the questions listed in Display 5-2.

Key Points   Implementation

1. *Implementation* involves the following activities:

   ☐ Continuing assessment and data collection

   ☐ Setting daily priorities

   ☐ Performing nursing interventions (see Guidelines: Performing Nursing Interventions)

   ☐ Documenting nursing care (see Guidelines: Charting Nurses' Notes)

   (continued)

☐ Giving verbal nursing reports (see Guidelines: Giving a Change-of-Shift Report)

☐ Maintaining a current care plan

2. Planning gives direction to implementation, but prescribed interventions are performed only when appropriate, as indicated by ongoing data collection.

3. Your ability to set daily priorities will depend upon your nursing knowledge and expertise, and your knowledge of routines at the facility where you work.

4. How you prioritize problems on a daily basis will be influenced by change-of-shift reports and assessment of medical and nursing records, but you must also take the time to verify this information by *direct patient assessment*.

5. The acronym "cwipat" can be used to remind you of the common tasks that should be accomplished before performing any nursing intervention. "Cwipat" stands for the following:

C = Check the orders and equipment.

W = Wash your hands.

I = *I*dentify the patient.

P = *P*rovide for safety and privacy.

A = *A*ssess the problem.

T = *T*ell the person or *T*each the person about what you're going to do.

6. The verbal reports that you give concerning your patient can have a major influence on the overall healthcare that he receives.

7. Charting is a legal requirement of all healthcare institutions: Poor (illegible, irrelevant, or incomplete) charting may impede care, while good (factual, descriptive, relevant) charting will communicate the pertinent aspects of the client's healthcare and help others to assess patterns of client responses.

8. Nursing care plans are useless unless they are kept up-to-date.

9. Part of the implementation phase includes ongoing evaluation of *both your patient and yourself*.

Bibliography

American Nurses' Association (1973) *Standards of Nursing Practice*, Kansas City, MO.

Burke, L. and Murphy, J. (1988) *Charting by Exception*. New York: John Wiley & Sons.

Carpenito, L. (1987) *Nursing Diagnosis: Application to Clinical Practice*. 2nd ed. Philadelphia: JB Lippincott.

Doering, K. and LaMountain, P. (1984) Flowcharts to facilitate caring for ostomy patients. *Nursing* 14(11):54–57.

Eggland, E. (1980) Charting: How and when to document your daily care. *Nursing '80* 10:38–43.

Gawlinski, A. and Rasmussen, S. (1984) Improving documentation through the use of change theory. *Focus* 11(6):12–17.

Gordon, M. (1982) *Nursing Diagnosis: Process and Application*. New York: McGraw-Hill.

Griffith, J. and Christensen, P. (1985) *Nursing Process: Application of Theories, Frameworks and Models*. St. Louis: CV Mosby.

Kerr, A. (1975) Nurses' notes: That's where the goodies are. *Nursing '75* 5:34–41.

Omdahl, D. (1988) Home care charting do's and don't's. *Am J. Nurs.* 88 (2):203–204.

Rich, P. (1983) Make the most of your charting time. *Nursing* 13(3):34–39.

Riegel, B. (1985) A method of giving intershift report based on a conceptual

☑ Establishing Outcome Criteria
☑ Evaluating Goal Achievement
☑ Identifying Variables Affecting Goal Achievement
☑ Modifying the Plan of Care/ Terminating Care

6
Evaluation

Standard VII: *The client's/patient's progress or lack of progress toward goal achievement is determined by the client/patient and the nurse.*

Standard VIII: *The client's/patient's progress or lack of progress toward goal achievement directs reassessment, reordering of priorities, new goal setting, and revision of the plan of nursing care.* *

*Abstracted from Standards of Nursing Practice. Copyright American Nurses' Association, 1973

Glossary

Nursing Audit A thorough investigation designed to examine a specific aspect of nursing care for the purpose of identifying and correcting problems, and establishing or examining standards of care.

Quality Assurance Activities and programs designed to identify and correct problems, and to set forth standards, protocols, policies, and procedures to guide nurses to give safe, effective, efficient nursing care.

Variable Factor that affects goal achievement positively (*e.g.*, good motivation) or negatively (*e.g.*, poor motivation).

Determining How Well the Plan Worked/ Making Changes/Terminating

You have completed assessment, diagnosis, planning, and implementation and are now ready for evaluation where you will determine how well the plan worked, and make changes or terminate interventions. Although you have begun early evaluation during the preceding steps of the nursing process by monitoring patient responses to interventions and by making necessary changes in the plan of care, it is during this step that you must complete thorough reassessment of the entire plan of care. This chapter presents the "how to's" of the following activities of the evaluation phase:

☐ Establishing the criteria for evaluation (outcome criteria)

☐ Evaluating goal achievement

☐ Assessing variables affecting goal achievement

☐ Modifying the plan of care/terminating nursing care

It will also discuss the need for providing quality assurance.

Establishing the Criteria for Client Goal Evaluation

Ideally, the criteria that you establish for evaluation of client goals will be the same as the goals or outcomes that you have identified on the care plan. That is, you established goals for your client during the planning phase, and now you must decide how well he has achieved the goals. Some institutions will have standards that list pre-established outcome criteria for certain problems/ diagnoses. Given that you have established goals that were congruent with these standards, the criteria for evaluation will be the goals that you established during planning.

Evaluating Client Goal Achievement

Evaluating client goal achievement begins with assessment. This means that you will have to examine and interview the patient, and gather data to determine his current health status and to answer the following questions:

☐ Are the problems the same as originally defined?

☐ Are they more complicated than originally described?

☐ Have new problems arisen?

Having answered the above questions, you now must ask,

☐ Are we ready to test goal achievement?

In some cases your initial assessment may tell you that you have been unable to meet your goals, and that it would be useless (even unsafe) to test goal achievement at this point. However, if you determine that the patient *is* ready to test goal achievement, then you would use appropriate techniques of assessment to gather the necessary information. If you are testing a patient behavior or activity (*e.g.*, ability to ambulate) you need to *compare your patient's behavior or ability to perform the activity (ambulate) with the established outcome criteria.* If it is a physical characteristic that you are trying to achieve (*e.g.*, good skin integrity), then you *compare your patient's physical characteristics* (*e.g.*, status of the skin) *with the desired characteristics that you described as outcome criteria* (*e.g.*, Is his skin intact and free from signs of irritation?).

Here is an example of the types of questions that you will be asking to determine goal achievement for the following goal: "Will walk half a mile in 10 minutes by 7/28."

☐ On 7/28, can the client walk a half a mile in 10 minutes?

☐ If he can, can he do it quite easily?

☐ If not, how far *can* he walk in 10 minutes?

☐ Is he close to his goal?

☐ Can he identify some factors that are affecting his ability to meet this goal?

Display 6-1 offers suggested steps for evaluating goal achievement.

Display 6-1. Steps for Evaluating Client Goal Achievement

1. Assess the client and determine whether he is ready to test for goal achievement. If he is, then proceed with Steps 2–8.

(continued)

2. List the goals (outcome criteria) that you have set forth in the planning phase.

    EXAMPLE:

    "Will walk unassisted the length of the hall by 7/3."

3. Assess what the client is able to do in relation to the goals.

    EXAMPLE:

    "Can walk unassisted the length of the hall, but he becomes a little unsteady toward the end of the walk."

4. Compare what the client is able to do with what you have set as his goal and ask the following questions:

    Has the goal been *completely* met? Can the client do *everything* set forth by the goal with the conditions set forth by the goal? How *well* does he perform the activities set forth by the goal?

    Has the goal been *partially* met? Is the client able to do only some of the activities set forth by the goal? Is he able to do the activities, but not with good proficiency? Does the client seem to be struggling to achieve the goal?

5. Discuss the goals with the client. Encourage him to verbalize his feelings about whether or not he has achieved the goals.

6. If all the goals have been easily achieved, are you moving too slowly, or are you going at just the right pace? Could you be doing more? Discuss this with the client, his family, and the healthcare team.

7. If the goals have been only partially met, or not met at all, gather data to determine what has gone wrong.

    Have short-term goals been met?

    Are the goals realistic for this individual?

    Does the client feel these goals are important?

    What does the client feel is important?

    Can the client identify anything that he feels may be slowing him down?

    Can you identify anything that may be slowing him down?

    Has the plan of care indeed been implemented, or have some actions been omitted?

8. Record your findings. Write an evaluation statement that includes how well goals have been achieved. (This is usually written in the column marked "evaluation" or "progress report" on the nursing care plan.)

☐ *Practice Session*   *Evaluating Client Goal Achievement*
(Suggested Answers on page 179)

For each number below, compare the outcome criteria with the listed observable patient data. Circle "A" if the goal has been achieved. Circle "P" if the goal has only been *partially* met. Circle "N" if the goal has *not* been met.

1. **Outcome Criteria:** Will demonstrate self-insulin injection, using aseptic technique.
   Observable Data: Injected self using good technique, but contaminated needle without noticing it.
   Answer: A P N

2. **Outcome Criteria:** Will demonstrate safe crutch walking, including climbing, and descending stairs.
   Observable Data: Demonstrates ability to use crutches for walking, climbing, and descending without problems.
   Answer: A P N

3. **Outcome Criteria:** Will relate the effect of increased exercise upon insulin demand.
   Observable Data: States that insulin demand is not affected by increased exercise.
   Answer: A P N

4. **Outcome Criteria:** Will maintain good skin integrity, free from signs of irritation.
   Observable Data: Skin is intact with some reddened areas noted on both elbows.
   Answer: A P N

5. **Outcome Criteria:** Will list the signs and symptoms of infection.
   Observable Data: Lists pain, swelling, and drainage.
   Answer: A P N

Identifying Variables Affecting Goal Achievement

To identify the variables affecting goal achievement, you will have to examine what happened during Planning and Implementation and answer the following questions:

☐ Were the goals and interventions realistic and appropriate for this individual?

☐ Were the interventions implemented consistently as prescribed?

☐ Were new problems or adverse patient responses detected early enough to make appropriate changes in the plan of care?

Examination of client records, especially nurses' notes and care plan progress notes, is essential to determining variables that may have affected goal achievement. If the client is unavailable or unable to communicate, the client records may be your *only* method of determining what happened on a day-to-day basis.

The client himself and significant others will often be the key people who will identify factors that have helped or hindered goal achievement. Sometimes these factors are so subtle that they will be identified only by those who know the client well, and by those who have been closely involved during implementation of the plan. The time you spend helping the client and other involved individuals to identify factors that they feel helped or hindered progress will be invaluable when you are modifying the plan of care, and later when you encounter future patients in similar situations.

You will have to apply your theoretical and practical knowledge to identify factors that may have affected goal achievement. For complicated situations, you should consider evaluating the plan of care in conference with all key members of the healthcare team, the patient and significant others, and an expert for additional insight.

Modifying the Plan of Care

Once you have determined whether you have set realistic goals and identified some variables that may be affecting goal achievement, you are now ready to modify the plan of care. You may need to establish new goals, identify new interventions, or change the environment or timing of interventions. Your ability to modify the plan of care and to make the necessary changes (to be realistic and to incorporate factors that enhance goal achievement and reduce or eliminate factors that deter progress) will be the key to achieving an efficient, effective, *individualized* plan of care.

Display 6-2 lists suggested steps to help you to modify your plan of care.

Terminating Nursing Care

If the client has achieved all the established goals and you have not identified new problems, you have achieved the ultimate aim of nursing care: terminating the plan of care and allowing the person full control over his own health. When you know you are ready to terminate nursing care, you can feel as though you and the patient have really met with success. Even though the actual act of terminating happens during the evaluation phase of the nursing process, terminating (or discharging) is something that you should be talking about from the time of your first encounter with the patient. During the entire time that you are delivering nursing care, you should be discussing "when you are discharged" whenever appropriate. This helps to prepare the patient from the beginning that the whole goal of nursing care should be that of making him as independent as possible.

Terminating nursing care involves a full assessment of how the patient plans to manage his health on his own. Display 6-3 on page 162 gives an example of the types of questions that need to be asked in preparation for discharge.

Once you have determined how the patient will manage on his own, written and verbal instructions for treatments, medications, and activities should be given to the patient to take home. Signs and symptoms of any possible future problems should be discussed, written down, and given to the patient to take home. Important telephone numbers and services that are available to the patient should also be discussed and written down. The patient and his family should be able to verbalize the types of problems they should be

Display 6-2.   Steps for Modifying the Plan of Care

1. Gather data to determine if any new problems have arisen and if your original nursing diagnoses and collaborative problems are still appropriate. Look for gaps or incongruities in the original assessment data that were documented. Seek to fill in the gaps and clarify incongruous facts by performing a full reassessment of the client.

2. Delete nursing diagnoses and collaborative problems that are not appropriate. Add any that are new.

3. Examine your list of nursing diagnoses and collaborative problems and set new priorities if necessary.

4. If you decide that the diagnoses and problems that you have identified are accurate and current, examine each established goal and ask the following questions:

   Is each goal derived specifically for a separate nursing diagnosis or collaborative problem?

   Are the goals realistic for this individual?

   Is the time frame for goal achievement realistic?

   Do the goals reflect individual capabilities and preferences of the client?

6. Change those goals that are unrealistic. (Either determine a more realistic goal, or set a new time frame for goal achievement.) Change those goals that do not reflect the individual preferences of your client. (Rewrite the goals to reflect his individual capabilities and preferences.)

7. Delete goals that are inappropriate, and add new goals if new problems or diagnoses have been identified.

8. Examine the interventions that have been identified for each of the appropriate goals, and ask the following:

   Is the written plan of nursing interventions being put into action consistently?

   Do the interventions promote individual client strengths?

   Is the timing of interventions appropriate, or should they be rearranged?

   Is the environment conducive to performing the activities necessary for the interventions?

   Are the interventions producing the desired responses?

   What are some additional factors or interventions that might help to produce the desired response?

9. Change or delete interventions that are inappropriate, and add any new interventions that have been identified.

10. Incorporate factors that contribute to your client's successful goal achievement, and delete or minimize factors that may be impeding progress.

11. Set new target dates for reevaluation.

avoiding and preventing, the correct management of their specific problems, and the resources that they may be planning to use to improve their health. Most healthcare facilities have their own discharge planning and discharge instruction forms that must be completed before discharge, and you should become familiar with each of these.

Display 6-3.   Discharge Planning Questionnaire

1. Is there a problem at home with any of the following?

Heat	Yes	No	Possibly
Hot/cold water	Yes	No	Possibly
Electricity	Yes	No	Possibly
Refrigeration	Yes	No	Possibly
Cooking Facilities	Yes	No	Possibly
Bathroom Facilities	Yes	No	Possibly

2. Is necessary transportation available?   Yes   No   Possibly

3. Can the person be reached by phone?   Yes   No   Possibly

   If no, is there a neighbor who can be reached by phone?   Yes   No   Possibly

4. Will the patient/family require:

Assistance with ADL	Yes	No	Possibly
Assistance with medications	Yes	No	Possibly
Assistance with treatments	Yes	No	Possibly
Additional teaching	Yes	No	Possibly
Ongoing nursing assessment	Yes	No	Possibly
Community resources or referrals	Yes	No	Possibly

The following diagram, reproduced from Chapter 1, summarizes the activities for evaluating goal achievement.

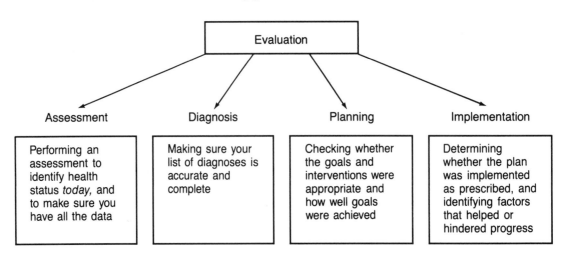

Evaluation			
Assessment	**Diagnosis**	**Planning**	**Implementation**
Performing an assessment to identify health status *today*, and to make sure you have all the data	Making sure your list of diagnoses is accurate and complete	Checking whether the goals and interventions were appropriate and how well goals were achieved	Determining whether the plan was implemented as prescribed, and identifying factors that helped or hindered progress

Providing Quality Assurance

It would be inappropriate to write a chapter on evaluation and not include its role in providing for quality assurance. That is, *evaluation is the key* for determining standards, protocols, policies, and procedures that will assist nurses to provide *quality nursing care.*

Providing for quality assurance involves *evaluating specific aspects of the nursing care of a group of patients in similar situations (or with similar problems).* Those of you who are beginners will be involved mostly in evaluating the care of an individual patient. However, you should be aware of the efforts of nurses and committees who perform audits to evaluate the care of groups of patients because it will be these types of projects that will provide the information to develop standards of care for the future. Through use of the evaluation process, nurses can take an active part in identifying common problems, determining methods to prevent their occurrence, and setting forth standards, protocols, policies, and procedures that will guide nurses in providing safe, efficient, and effective nursing care.

Key Points   Evaluation

1. The fifth step of the nursing process, evaluation, involves a complete reassessment of the entire plan of nursing care.

2. Evaluation involves the following activities:
   □ Establishing outcome criteria
   □ Assessing current patient status
   □ Evaluating goal achievement
   □ Determining variables affecting goal achievement
   □ Modifying plan of care/terminating nursing care

3. Whether a goal has been achieved should be determined by both the client and the nurse.

4. To determine client goal achievement, you must ascertain what the client can do in relation to the goals set forth during the planning phase of the nursing process.

5. Evaluation involves assessing what factors may be contributing to the success of the plan, and what factors may be impeding

progress. Without accurate documentation, the only sources of this information may be the memories of the patient, family, and nurse.

6. Modifying the plan of care involves revising it to reflect the necessary changes that were noted by full reassessment of the nursing care plan.

7. Terminating nursing care, or discharge planning, should begin as early in the plan of care as possible. For example, when appropriate, include discussions of "when you are discharged" even if the discharge date is a long way off.

8. Providing quality assurance involves studying specific aspects of a group of patients with similar problems (or in similar situations) for the purpose of developing standards, protocols, or procedures that can guide the nurse to provide safe, efficient, effective nursing care.

Bibliography

American Nurses' Association (1973) *Standards of Nursing Practice*. Kansas City, MO.

Block, D. (1977) Criteria, standards, norms—crucial terms in quality assurance. *J. Nurs. Adm.* 7(9):20–30.

Carpenito, L. (1987) *Nursing Diagnosis: Application to Clinical Practice*. 2nd ed. Philadelphia: JB Lippincott.

Chow, R. (1978) Assuring the quality of care: A personal perspective—from tailoring to outcome measurement. *Nurs. Leadersh.* 1(3):11–22.

Duke University Hospital Nursing Services. (1983) *Duke Guidelines for Nursing Care: Process and Outcome*. 2nd ed. Philadelphia: JB Lippincott.

Hover, J. and Zimmer, M. (1978) Nursing quality assurance: The Wisconsin system. *Nurs. Outlook* 26:242–248.

Hushower, G., Gamberg, D., and Smith, N. (1978) The nursing process in discharge planning. *Supervisor Nurse* 9(9):55–58.

Mayers, M., Norby, R., and Watson, A. (1976) *Quality Assurance for Patient Care: Nursing Perspectives*. New York: Appleton-Century-Crofts.

Phaneuf, M. (1976) *The Nursing Audit: Self-Regulation in Nursing Practice*. New York: Appleton-Century-Crofts.

Roeder, M. (1978) Patient care plans and the evaluation of the nursing process. *Supervisor Nurse* 11(1):57–58.

Sanborn, C. and Blount, M. (1984) Standard plans for care and discharge. *Am. J. Nurs.* (11):1394–1396.

Warren, J. (1981) Accountability and nursing diagnosis. *J. Nurs. Adm.* 13:34–37.

Suggested Answers to Practice Sessions

Note

When you check your answers with the answers on the following pages, please remember that these are *suggested* answers. In some cases, you may find that you have somewhat different answers than the suggested answers. This does not necessarily mean that your answer is wrong. It is difficult to present a clear, concise case history on paper—too often there is room for varied interpretation by the reader. These sessions are meant to *provide practice* in the thinking process necessary to complete the steps of the nursing process, and these are the *suggested* answers, not the *only* answers. Check with your instructor if you have a question.

Chapter 1: Nursing Process Overview *(page 9)*

1. **Assessment:** Gathering and examining data for the purpose of identifying actual and potential health problems
   Diagnosis: Analyzing data and pulling it together to identify the exact nature of a health problem
   Planning: Establishing goals and determining nursing interventions
   Implementation: Putting the plan into action
   Evaluation: Performing an assessment, checking the diagnoses, measuring goal achievement, determining factors that influenced patient care, and terminating or modifying the plan of care as indicated

2. The nursing process plan focuses on *human responses,* while the medical treatment plan focuses on *disease.* The nursing process plan is more likely to change on a day-to-day basis as human responses change. The medical treatment plan is more likely to stay the same for longer periods of time. The nursing process also deals more with families and groups than does the average medical treatment plan.

3. Provides for organized nursing care

   Prevents omissions and unnecessary repetitions

   Provides for better communication

   Focuses on the individual's unique human response and complements medical treatment plan

   Promotes flexibility in giving individualized nursing care

   Encourages participation on the part of the patient/family and utilizes strengths

   Helps nurses to gain satisfaction by getting results

4. *Keeping an eye closely focused on individual/family experiences and perceptions* will help you to make a plan of care that is *realistic and efficient.* Including patients and families in making decisions and developing a plan of care helps to assure that the person who can offer some of the most significant data (*i.e.,* the patient) has input in developing the plan of care.

Chapter 2: Assessment

The Nursing Interview *(page 31)*

1. Making open-ended questions
   a. "Describe how you feel."
   b. "How was your dinner?"
   c. "How does being here make you feel?"
   d. "Describe what it feels like."
   e. "Tell me about your relationship with your wife."

2. Clarifying ideas by using reflection and making open-ended questions

   a. "You've been sick off and on for a month? Describe what the sickness is like."

   b. "Nothing ever goes right for you? Give some examples of what you mean."

   c. "So, you have a pain in your side that is intermittent. Explain how it feels and what you mean by 'comes and goes.'"

   d. " . . . A funny feeling? Describe the feeling."

   e. "You feel weak all over? Give me some examples of things that make you feel weak."

The Nursing Physical Assessment (page 34)

1. a. "You have a lot of ground-in dirt here. What's this from?"

   b. "I feel a lump on the back of your head. How did it happen? Does it hurt when I touch it?"

   c. "Your breathing is a little fast. How does it feel?"

   d. "Your eye seems inflamed. How does it feel?"

   e. "I see you have some cavities. When did you last go to the dentist?"

2. a. "Show me where" (and examine that area).

   b. "Show me where" (and examine that area).

   c. "That's a common symptom of infection. Let's get a urine specimen" (and examine it).

   d. "Where have you felt this bloated feeling . . . your stomach, ankles, where?" Examine that specific area, extremities, abdomen, and auscultate heart and lungs.

   e. "Show me where" (and examine that area).

3. **Case History A**

   a. Mental status

      Vital signs

      Pain

      Fluid and electrolyte balance

   b. Interview Mrs. Laird about symptoms/concerns.

      Ask about abdominal symptoms (pain, nausea, vomiting, bowel movements).

      Perform abdominal assessment. (Assess for presence of bowel sounds, distention, tenderness.)

      Assess fluid intake and output. (Assess for dehydration.)

      Read medical and nursing records (care plan, nurses' notes, progress notes, lab studies, x-ray reports).

Case History B

   c. Vital signs

       Respiratory status (lung sounds, cough, mucus production, whether he has been smoking since surgery, method for coughing)

       Surgical incision/heparin lock

       When last analgesic was administered

       Assess fluid intake and output. (Assess for adequate hydration.)

   d. Interview Mr. Daniels about symptoms/concerns.

       Perform an abdominal assessment. Examine incision.

       Auscultate lungs.

       Have the patient demonstrate coughing and deep breathing (examine sputum).

       Read medical and nursing records (care plan, nurses' notes, progress reports, lab studies, x-ray reports).

Subjective and Objective Data *(page 36)*

Case History A

1. 51 years old

   No pain

   Feels better

   Feels relieved

2. Lab study results

   Talking slowly

   Frequent sighing

   Vital signs

Case History B

1. 33 years old

   Mother of two

   "I can't believe I have diabetes."

   "I don't think I can change my eating habits."

   Feels fine, but tired lately

   Increased urination

2. Weight: 190 lb

   Blood sugar: 144

   Vital signs

Identifying Cues and Making Inferences *(page 38)*

1. a. All the subjective and objective data listed under Mr. Michaels in the previous practice session

b. Physical condition improving

Seems depressed

2. a. All the subjective and objective data listed under Mrs. Rochester in the previous practice session

b. Seems reluctant to admit she has diabetes

Seems anxious concerning effects of diabetes and changes in life-style (*e.g.*, eating habits)

May be angry about diagnosis

Validating Assessment Data (page 40)

1. a.

Certainly Valid	*Probably Valid*	*Possibly Valid*
Lab studies	51 years old	Feels relieved
Talking slowly	No pain	
Frequent sighing	Feels better	
	Vital signs	

b. Compare stated age with birthdate.

Ask probing questions to describe comfort state (*e.g.*, "Are you *sure* you don't have any discomfort at all?").

Observe for nonverbal signs of discomfort (*e.g.*, rubbing hand on chest).

Spend quality time with Mr. Michaels discussing how he feels physically and psychologically.

Recheck vital signs if you are concerned that they are inaccurate.

2. a.

Certainly Valid	*Probably Valid*	*Possibly Valid*
Weight: 190 lb	33 years old	Angry about having diabetes
Blood sugar: 144	Mother of two	May be denying that she has diabetes
	Anxious	
	Feels tired	
	Increased urination	

b. Compare stated age with birthdate.

Measure time and amount of urine output.

Spend quality time discussing feelings and concerns about changes in life-style.

Organizing Assessment Data (page 46)

1. **Case History A**

If you used Maslow's hierarchy of needs:

Physiological needs: 5,6,7,9,11,12,13,14

Safety/security needs: 10

Love and belonging needs: 2,4,8

Self-esteem needs: 3,8,11,13

Self-actualization needs: 3

Case History B

If you used Gordon's functional health patterns:

Health-perception–health-management pattern: 10,11

Nutritional-metabolic pattern: 1,5,6,9,13,14,16

Elimination pattern: 9

Activity/exercise pattern: 2

Cognitive-perceptual pattern: 12

Sleep-rest pattern: 8

Self-perception–self-concept pattern: 1,2,3

Role-relationship pattern: 2,3,7

Sexuality-reproductive pattern: 1,2

Coping-stress-tolerance pattern: 7,12

Value-belief pattern: 4

2. **Case History A:** 5,6,7,9,10,12,13,14

   Case History B: 5,6,8,9,10,13,15

Chapter 3: Diagnosis

Identifying Signs and Symptoms *(page 64)*

1. a. nl   f. nl
   b. abnl   g. abnl
   c. nl   h. abnl
   d. abnl   i. nl
   e. abnl   j. abnl

2. a. 0   f. 0
   b. si   g. sy
   c. 0   h. si
   d. si   i. 0
   e. si   j. si

Nursing Diagnoses and Collaborative Problems (page 68)

1. CP	6. ND	11. CP
2. ND	7. CP	12. ND
3. ND	8. CP	13. ND
4. CP	9. ND	14. CP
5. ND	10. CP	15. CP

Using the PES Format (page 71)

1. Impaired Gas Exchange related to smoking as manifested by chronic cough productive of mucus, constant smoking, elevated CO_2

2. Altered Nutrition: Less Than Body Requirements related to loss of appetite as manifested by 10-lb weight loss and weight that is 15 lb less than the recommended weight

3. Impaired Physical Mobility related to inability to move lower limbs as manifested by inability to move both lower legs and limited passive range of motion in lower joints

Writing Diagnostic Statements for Potential and Possible Nursing Diagnoses (page 73)

1. Possible Ineffective Individual Coping related to problems with his girl-friend and possibly related to confinement to bed

2. Potential Fluid Volume Deficit related to insufficient fluid intake

3. Potential Ineffective Airway Clearance related to history of smoking and recent general anesthesia

4. Possible Sexual Dysfunction possibly related to recent hysterectomy, or possibly related to poor relationship with her husband

Identifying Correctly Stated Nursing Diagnoses (page 80)

The following are correct: 1, 5, 6, 8, 9, 13, 15

Identifying Nursing Diagnoses and Collaborative Problems (page 83)

Case History A (Mrs. Goode)

Strengths:

Normal vital signs

Moves all extremities with equal strength, strong peripheral pulses, abdomen soft, equal pupils

Nursing Diagnoses:

Potential for Injury related to dizziness

Potential Altered Patterns of Urinary Elimination related to inability to use bed pan

Fear related to hospitalization as manifested by statements of fear of hospitals and needles

Possible Altered Family Processes related to Mrs. Goode's illness

Collaborative Problems:

Potential Complication: increased intracranial pressure secondary to concussion

Potential Complication: phlebitis or tissue injury at intravenous site

Case History B (Mr. Northe)

Strengths:

Satisfactory peripheral pulses/good circulation

Nursing Diagnoses:

Constipation related to inactivity as manifested by no bowel movement in 5 days

Impaired Physical Mobility related to prescribed bedrest as manifested by prescribed bedrest

Potential Ineffective Individual Coping related to prescribed bedrest

Possible Fear of Death related to brother's death under the same circumstances

Possible Spiritual Distress related to uncertainty of cardiac condition and threat to life

Impaired Skin Integrity as manifested by red pressure areas on both heels

Collaborative Problems:

Potential Complications:

Cardiac arrhythmias

Congestive heart failure secondary to possible myocardial infarction

Pulmonary edema

Oliguria

Fluid overload per IV

Phlebitis, tissue injury at IV site

Chapter 4: Planning

Setting Priorities (page 94)

1. (a) immediate (b) nursing care plan (c) referred

2. The whole picture of the patient's problems.

   Patient's perception of what is important

   The overall plan of care

   The presence of potential problems

   The overall health status of the patient

3. b

4. a. N
   b. R
   c. R
   d. N
   e. R

Writing Client Goals/Outcomes for Nursing Diagnoses (page 102)

1. List, identify, describe, verbalize, demonstrate, report

2. The following are *incorrect:*

   a. The verb is not measurable.

   c. Nonspecific. How will we measure what is meant by "will improve?"

   f. No time criterion. Verb is not measurable and observable.

   h. No time criterion. Verb is not measurable and observable.

   j. Verb is not measurable.

3. a. After increasing roughage intake, Mrs. Pierce will report having one soft, formed bowel movement every 1 to 2 days, beginning Thursday.

   b. After Diane begins performing daily tooth brushing, flossing, and gum care, her gums will be pink and healthy looking (by 10/28).

   c. When observed, the skin around Mr. Culp's incision will be clean, with no signs of redness or irritation.

   d. After instruction, Mrs. Sovosky will correctly express needs by using flash cards (by 4/26).

   e. After a visit by the chaplain, Heidi will verbalize that it is "OK with God" if she is unable to go to daily Mass and that knowing this makes her feel more peaceful.

   f. Mrs. O'Dell will demonstrate how to feed herself with the use of padded spoons by 5/9.

   g. Mr. Noll will stop smoking or reduce smoking and/or report to the nurse if he develops respiratory symptoms.

   h. Mrs. Bell will eat three balanced meals every day with a caloric intake of 2000.

   i. Mr. Roberts will not be disturbed, but will be observed sleeping soundly for periods of 4 hours at night beginning tonight.

   j. Jane will report ability to void at least 200 ml without pain or urgency.

Domains of Expected Outcomes *(page 106)*

1. a. Cognitive and psychomotor
   b. Cognitive
   c. Affective
   d. Cognitive
   e. Cognitive and psychomotor
   f. Psychomotor
   g. Affective
   h. Psychomotor and cognitive
   i. Cognitive
   j. Cognitive, psychomotor, and affective

2. a. View film on infant nutrition and formula feedings on 4/5.

   Describe the steps involved in preparing and sterilizing formula on 4/5.

   Demonstrate preparing and sterilizing baby formula on 4/6.

   b. Read the procedure for sterilization, and clarify any questions with primary nurse on 5/1.

   Verbalize the reasons for sterilization on 5/10.

   c. Discuss with primary nurse on 2/2 how patient feels about going home.

   d. Attend the diabetic class on nutrition on 10/11.

   Discuss with primary nurse the relationship between blood sugar levels and eating certain foods on 10/11.

   Review printed diet restrictions on 10/12.

   e. Attend the group diabetic class on insulin administration and monitoring of blood sugar levels on 7/28.

   View teaching filmstrips on insulin administration and the monitoring of blood sugar on 7/29.

   Observe the nurse demonstrating the correct procedures for insulin administration and for testing blood sugar level on 7/30.

   Practice insulin self-administration based on morning blood sugar readings beginning 7/31.

   f. After instruction by physical therapy on 12/2, Mr. Roberts will begin practicing walking with a cane, gradually increasing how far he walks until he can walk the length of the hall (by 12/7).

   g. On 1/14 discuss with Mrs. Bell the importance of verbalizing when she is worried or concerned.

   h. On 3/2, have Debbie observe the correct technique for postural drainage, then encourage her to ask questions for clarification.

On 3/3 and 3/4 have Debbie practice performing postural drainage under close supervision.

i. Teach Matt the signs and symptoms of hypoglycemia using the "diabetic game" on 2/5.

Informally quiz Matt on the signs and symptoms on 2/6, and reinforce information that he does not seem to know.

j. Watch film on balanced nutrition on 11/11.

Discuss how Jimmy can make time to cook and eat breakfast.

Assist Jimmy to incorporate favorite foods into a balanced diet.

Determining Nursing Interventions for Nursing Diagnoses (page 114)

1. Assess skin integrity, especially over bony prominences, with each position change.

   Assess protein and vitamin C intake.

   Develop (and post at bedside) a q 2 hr turning schedule that enlists the client's maximal participation.

   Massage bony prominences with Alpha Keri lotion with position changes, and document daily appearance of skin.

   Keep an air mattress on the bed. Keep sheets clean, dry, and unwrinkled.

2. **Preoperatively:**

   After demonstrating the correct procedure for coughing and deep breathing with incisional splinting, assess the patient's and family's knowledge of these procedures via return demonstration.

   Postoperatively:

   Assess for incisional pain. Medicate p.r.n. as indicated and chart effect.

   Auscultate lungs bilaterally, and record findings.

   Assist client with coughing and deep breathing q 2 hr the day of surgery and first postoperative day.

   Teach the client the importance of position changes, early ambulation, and coughing and deep breathing.

3. Continue to monitor daily bowel habits and keep a record of bowel movements.

   Teach the client the relationship between exercise, diet, fluid intake, and normal bowel elimination.

   Develop with the client a specific plan for gradually increasing daily activity (*e.g.*, using stairs instead of elevator, or walking briskly) and for increasing dietary intake of roughage and fluids (especially water).

4. Assess incisional dressing with each postoperative change.

   When changing the dressing, assess the incision for signs of healing. Report any signs of infection: redness, swelling, drainage with foul odor.

Utilize sterile technique when changing the dressing: cleanse the incision with betadine and cover with a sterile dressing.

Document dressing changes and assessment findings.

Teach the client how to care for the healing incision at home, including how to detect and manage complications.

5. Primary nurse should discuss with client key factors of his hospitalization that are making the client feel powerless.

Determine with client what aspects of his hospitalization he feels that he is able to control

Alert the nursing staff to give client control in as many of these areas as possible.

Teach the client that his body and his health are his own and that he has the right to make autonomous decisions about his healthcare. Provide the knowledge base that makes this possible. Support him in physician–client interactions.

Monitoring to Detect Potential Complications *(page 117)*

1. **Potential Complications:** Infiltration, phlebitis, thrombus formation, fluid overload, infection.

   Plan for monitoring to detect potential complications: Follow hospital policy/standard. Monitor vital signs q 4 hr. Check IV site for signs and symptoms of infection, infiltration, phlebitis, thrombus q 4 hr. Check IV rate q hr. Document intake and output q 8 hr. Instruct the patient to notify you if the IV becomes uncomfortable.

2. **Potential Complications:** Hypoglycemia/hyperglycemia.

   Plan for monitoring to detect potential complications: Follow hospital policy/standard. Monitor caloric intake at each meal. Monitor blood sugar via glucometer q 6 hr. Instruct the patient to notify nurses if dizziness or apprehension is experienced.

3. **Potential Complications:** Infection, blockage of the catheter.

   Plan for monitoring to detect potential complications: Follow hospital policy/standard. Monitor temperature q 4–8 hr. Check urine output q 4 hr for color, sediment, amount. Document intake and output q 8 hr. Check insertion site q 8 hr for drainage. Instruct the patient to notify you if the catheter feels uncomfortable.

Writing Nursing Orders *(page 121)*

1. Develop a turning schedule for q 2 hr position changes and post the schedule at bedside.

Assess the client's understanding of the need for position changes and ability/willingness to help. Assess the family's ability/desire to assist with position changes.

Turn the client q 2 hr, noting any changes in skin integrity, massaging bony prominences, and providing for good body alignment.

2. Assess what fluid preferences the client has and order these fluids for the unit. Keep preferred fluids at the bedside at all times.

    Utilize all client interactions to encourage fluid intake. Each shift should be responsible for

    7–3 = 1800 ml   3–11 = 1000 ml   11–7 = 200 ml

    Teach the client the importance of increasing his fluid intake. Assess his understanding of the need to force fluids and his willingness to do so.

    Tell the person the goal for fluid intake and have him record what he drinks.

    Document intake and output q shift.

3. Utilize all patient interactions (nursing rounds, bath time, treatments, *etc.*) to develop a trusting nurse–patient relationship. Utilize empathic behaviors that express genuine caring.

    Encourage the person to express her feelings by using open-ended questions (*e.g.*, "It must be hard to lie there all afternoon with nothing to do but think. What are you thinking about?").

    If one or more nurses establish a good rapport with this patient, assign them frequently to her care.

    Attempt to determine why it is difficult for this individual to express her feelings. Share with her the positive benefits of expression, as well as the potential negative consequences of holding things in.

4. Assess the client's normal pattern of bowel elimination. Note any stimuli to bowel elimination (*e.g.*, jogging, morning coffee, *etc.*)

    Teach the client the relationship between adequate fluid/roughage intake and exercise and regular bowel elimination.

    Teach the client the negative consequences of repeatedly ignoring the urge to defecate.

    Teach the client the harmful effects of prolonged use of laxatives and enemas.

    Instruct the client to record his daily bowel elimination, noting diet, exercise, and use of laxatives.

    Document color and character of stools.

5. Assist patient out of bed to chair for a half hour, at 10 A.M. and 8 P.M. Provide two pillows for his back, and stool for feet. Leave call bell attached to arm of chair.

Chapter 5: Implementation

Charting Nurses' Notes *(page 146)*

Case A (Mr. Johns)

Date and Time	Of Special Notation	Nursing Assessment and Comments
11/22/90		
8:30 AM		Sitting OOB in chair. Seems to be wheezing more than usual—using accessory muscles of the chest. Denies increased difficulty breathing.
8:40 AM	Reg $\frac{170}{94}$ 97–130–30	Respiratory rate unchanged, but he is more restless & confused (doesn't know he's in the hospital). _____ J. LeFevre, RN
8:45 AM	O$_2$ started @ 2 liters/min per cannula	Assisted back to bed. Siderails ↑ ._____ Still wheezing and appears in distress. Dr. Payne notified. _____ J. LeFevre, RN
9 AM	Exam by Dr. Payne	Condition unchanged. _____ J. LeFevre, RN
9:10 AM	ABGs drawn by Lab	Pressure to puncture site applied for 5 minutes—no bleeding. _____ J. LeFevre, RN
9:15 AM	Resp Therapist here for IPPB Rx. _____	Coughed up large amounts of thick white mucus. _____ J. LeFevre, RN
9:35 AM		Lungs more clear. He is no longer confused. Able to take a few sips of water. J. LeFevre, RN Much improved. Assisted OOB to chair.
10 AM	P-110 R-28	_____ J. LeFevre, RN

Case B (Mrs. Fox)

Date and Time	Of Special Notation	Nursing Assessment and Comments
6/14/90 5 PM		Assisted to give her own insulin. _____ She contaminated needle and did not notice it. Reinforced the importance of maintaining sterile techniques. _____ J Koonce, RN
8 PM		Ate all of her dinner tonight, but she states that she is "dying for a chocolate bar"—she states that following a diabetic diet will be impossible. Discussed possibility of talking c̄ dietitian re: changes in diet. _____ J Koonce, RN
8:30 PM		Encouraged to do things to get her mind off of food. Called a friend to chat ____ J Koonce, RN
9 PM		Offered her fruit & milk snack—ate it all & drank milk. _____ J Koonce, RN
9:30–9:55		Spent time discussing her feelings about all the changes that she has to make because of diabetes. Is more optimistic now. ____ J Koonce, RN
10 PM		Resting quietly in bed. _____ J Koonce, RN

Chapter 6: Evaluation

Evaluating Goal Achievement *(page 157)*

1. P
2. A
3. N
4. N
5. P

QUICK REFERENCE TO NURSING DIAGNOSES

This section has been designed for quick retrieval of information for each of the nursing diagnostic categories accepted by NANDA for study and clinical testing. An alphabetical listing is followed by each category label's corresponding definition, defining characteristics, and related/contributing factors.

Most of the information comes directly from *NANDA Taxonomy I* (1987), with minor adaption by myself for clarification. An asterisk (*) has been placed whenever the information has been adapted. Changes approved by NANDA in 1988 are also included.

Though I personally find some of the diagnostic category labels to be problematic for use in the clinical setting, all accepted labels are included to provide a comprehensive listing.

I acknowledge and applaud the work of the nurses who have submitted and refined the category labels as described in *NANDA Taxonomy I*. However, since the work of refining and researching these category labels is not yet complete, I encourage those of you who identify new diagnoses (or diagnoses that are on the list, but need refinement) to communicate this information to NANDA (see "Requirements for Submitting a Proposed New Nursing Diagnosis," page 208).

(The complete *NANDA Taxonomy I* can be purchased by contacting NANDA at 3525 Caroline Street, St. Louis, MO 63104)

Alphabetical Listing of Nursing Diagnoses
(Includes all diagnoses accepted for study and clinical testing by NANDA as of 1988)

Activity Intolerance
Activity Intolerance, Potential
Adjustment, Impaired
Airway Clearance, Ineffective
Anxiety
Aspiration, Potential for†

Body Image Disturbance‡
Body Temperature, Potential Altered
Bowel Incontinence‡
Breastfeeding, Ineffective†
Breathing Pattern, Ineffective

---

† New diagnostic category approved by NANDA in 1988.

‡ Revised/modified by NANDA in 1988.

§ Author recommends adding this category label to the list.

Cardiac Output, Decreased‡
Communication, Impaired§
Communication, Impaired Verbal
Conflict, Decisional (Specify)†
Conflict, Parental Role†
Constipation‡
Constipation, Colonic†
Constipation, Perceived†
Coping, Defensive†
Coping, Family: Potential for Growth
Coping, Ineffective Family: Compromised
Coping, Ineffective Family: Disabling
Coping, Ineffective Individual

Denial, Ineffective
Diarrhea‡
Disuse, Potential for†
Diversional Activity Deficit
Dysreflexia†

Family Processes, Altered
Fatigue†
Fear
Fluid Volume Deficit, Actual
Fluid Volume Deficit, Potential
Fluid Volume Excess

Gas Exchange, Impaired
Grieving§
Grieving, Anticipatory
Grieving, Dysfunctional
Growth and Development, Altered

Health Maintenance, Altered
Health Seeking Behavior (Specify)†
Home Maintenance Management, Impaired
Hopelessness

Hyperthermia
Hypothermia‡

Infection, Potential for
Injury, Potential for

Knowledge Deficit (Specify)

Mobility, Impaired Physical

Noncompliance
Nutrition, Altered: Less Than Body
    Requirements
Nutrition, Altered: More Than Body
    Requirements
Nutrition, Altered: Potential for More Than
    Body Requirements

Oral Mucous Membrane, Altered‡

Pain‡
Pain, Chronic
Parenting, Altered
Parenting, Potential Altered
Personal Identity Disturbance
Poisoning, Potential for
Post-Trauma Response
Powerlessness

Rape-Trauma Syndrome
Rape-Trauma Syndrome: Compound Reaction
Rape-Trauma Syndrome: Silent Reaction
Role Performance, Altered‡

---

† New diagnostic category approved by NANDA in 1988.

‡ Revised/modified by NANDA in 1988.

§ Author recommends adding this category label to the list.

Self-Care Deficit, Bathing/Hygiene‡
Self-Care Deficit, Dressing/Grooming†
Self-Care Deficit, Feeding‡
Self-Care Deficit, Toileting‡
Self-Esteem Disturbance†‡
Self-Esteem, Chronic Low†
Self-Esteem, Situational Low†
Sensory/Perceptual Alterations (Specify): Visual, Auditory, Kinesthetic, Gustatory, Tactile, Olfactory
Sexual Dysfunction
Sexuality Patterns, Altered
Skin Integrity, Impaired
Skin Integrity, Potential Impaired
Sleep Pattern Disturbance
Social Interaction, Impaired
Social Isolation
Spiritual Distress
Suffocation, Potential for
Swallowing, Impaired

Thermoregulation, Ineffective
Thought Processes, Altered
Tissue Integrity, Impaired
Tissue Perfusion, Altered (Specify): Renal, Cerebral, Cardiopulmonary, Gastrointestinal, Peripheral‡
Trauma, Potential for

Unilateral Neglect
Urinary Elimination, Altered Patterns of‡
(Urinary) Incontinence, Functional†
(Urinary) Incontinence, Reflex†
(Urinary) Incontinence, Stress†
(Urinary) Incontinence, Total†
(Urinary) Incontinence, Urge†
Urinary Retention†

Violence, Potential for

---

† New diagnostic category approved by NANDA in 1988.

‡ Revised/modified by NANDA in 1988.

§ Author recommends adding this category label to the list.

Throughout, an asterisk (*) indicates that a section of the diagnosis has been adapted by the author. If no asterisk appears, the section is unchanged from NANDA Taxonomy I.

Activity Intolerance

(see also *Activity Intolerance, Potential; Breathing Pattern, Ineffective; Cardiac Output, Decreased; Fatigue*)

A state in which an individual has insufficient physiological or psychological energy to endure or complete required or desired daily activities.

Major Defining Characteristics

Verbal report of fatigue or weakness; abnormal heart rate or blood pressure response to activity; exertional discomfort or dyspnea; electrocardiographic changes reflecting arrhythmias or ischemia.

Related/Contributing Factors*

Bedrest/immobility; generalized weakness; sedentary lifestyle; imbalance between oxygen supply/demand; anemia; aging process; deconditioned state.

Activity Intolerance, Potential

(see also *Breathing Pattern, Ineffective; Cardiac Output, Decreased; Fatigue*)

A state in which an individual *is at risk* of experiencing insufficient physiological or psychological energy to endure or complete required or desired daily activities.

Defining Characteristics/Risk Factors

History of previous activity intolerance; deconditioned status; presence of circulatory/respiratory problems; inexperience with the activity.

Related/Contributing Factors*

Bedrest/immobility; generalized weakness; sedentary lifestyle; imbalance between oxygen supply/demand; anemia; aging process; deconditioned state.

*Adapted by author.

Adjustment, Impaired

(see also *Coping, Ineffective Individual*)

The state in which the individual is unable to modify his or her life-style/behavior in a manner consistent with a change in health status.

Major Defining Characteristics

Verbalization of nonacceptance of health status change; nonexistent or unsuccessful ability to be involved in problem-solving or goal-setting.

Minor Defining Characteristics

Lack of movement toward independence; extended period of shock, disbelief, or anger regarding health status change; lack of future-oriented thinking.

Related/Contributing Factors*

Disability requiring change in life-style; inadequate support systems; impaired cognition; sensory overload; assault to self-esteem; altered locus of control; incomplete grieving.

Airway Clearance, Ineffective

(see also *Aspiration, Potential for; Breathing Pattern, Ineffective; Gas Exchange, Impaired*)

A state in which an individual is unable to clear secretions or obstructions from the respiratory tract to maintain airway patency.

Major Defining Characteristics*

Abnormal breath sounds such as rales (crackles) or rhonchi (wheezes); changes in rate or depth of respiration; tachypnea; cough, effective/ineffective, with or without sputum; cyanosis; dyspnea; tachycardia; verbal report of fear of coughing.

Related/Contributing Factors*

Decreased energy/fatigue; tracheobronchial infection, obstruction, secretion; perceptual/cognitive impairment; trauma; incisional pain; fear of rupturing sutures; dehydration; anesthesia; intubation.

Anxiety

(see also *Fear*)

A vague uneasy feeling whose source is often nonspecific or unknown to the individual.

Major Defining Characteristics*

Subjective: increased tension; apprehension; painful and persistent increased helplessness; uncertainty; fearful; scared; regretful; overexcited; rattled; distressed; jittery; feelings of inadequacy; shakiness; fear of unspecific consequences; expressed concerns re change in life events; worried; anxious; fear of loss; verbal report of many life stressors.

Objective: sympathetic stimulation—cardiovascular excitation, superficial vasoconstriction, pupil dilation; restlessness; insomnia; glancing about; poor eye contact; trembling/hand tremors; extraneous movement (foot shuffling, hand/arm movements); facial tension; voice quivering; focus on "self"; increased wariness; increased perspiration.

Related/Contributing Factors

Unconscious conflict about essential values/goals of life; threat to self-concept; threat of death; threat to or change in health status; threat to or change in role functioning; threat to or change in environment; threat to or change in interaction patterns; situational/maturational crises; interpersonal transmission/contagion; unmet needs.

Aspiration, Potential for
(see also *Airway Clearance, Ineffective; Suffocation, Potential for*)

The state in which the individual is at risk for entry of gastrointestinal or oropharyngeal secretions, or solids or fluids into the tracheobronchial passages.

Defining Characteristics/Risk Factor*

Reduced level of consciousness; depressed cough and gag reflexes; presence of tracheostomy or endotracheal tube; incomplete lower esophageal sphincter; gastrointestinal tubes; tube feedings; medication administration; situations hindering elevation of upper body; increased intragastric pressure; increased gastric residual; decreased gastrointestinal motility; delayed gastric emptying; impaired swallowing; facial/oral/neck surgery or trauma; wired jaws.

Body Image Disturbance

Disruption in the way one perceives one's body image.

*Adapted by author.

Defining Characteristics

Objective: missing body part; actual change in structure and/or function; not looking at body part; not touching body part; hiding or overexposing body part (intentional or unintentional); trauma to nonfunctioning part; change in social involvement; change in ability to estimate spatial relationship of body to environment.

Subjective: verbalization of change in life-style; fear of rejection or of reaction by others; focus on past strength, function, or appearance; negative feelings about body; feelings of helplessness, hopelessness, or powerlessness; preoccupation with change or loss; emphasis on remaining strengths, heightened achievement; extension of body boundary to incorporate environmental objects; personalization of part or loss by name; depersonalization of part or loss by impersonal pronouns; refusal to verify actual change.

Related/Contributing Factors

Biophysical, cognitive/perceptual, psychosocial, cultural, or spiritual factors.

Body Temperature, Potential Altered
(see also *Hyperthermia; Hypothermia*)

The state in which the individual is at risk for failure to maintain body temperature within normal range.

Defining Characteristics/Risk Factors

Extremes of age; extremes of weight; exposure to cold/cool or warm/hot environments; dehydration; inactivity or vigorous activity; medications causing vasoconstriction/vasodilation; altered metabolic rate; sedation; inappropriate clothing for environmental temperature; illness or trauma affecting temperature regulation.

Bowel Incontinence
(see also *Diarrhea*)

A state in which an individual experiences a change in normal bowel habits characterized by involuntary passage of stool.

Major Defining Characteristic

Involuntary passage of stool.

Related/Contributing Factors*

Diarrhea; confusion; decreased level of conciousness; poor sphincter tone.

Breastfeeding, Ineffective

(see also *Parenting, Altered*)

The state in which a mother, infant, or child experiences dissatisfaction or difficulty with the breastfeeding process.

Major Defining Characteristics

Unsatisfactory breastfeeding process.

Minor Defining Characteristics

Actual or perceived inadequate milk supply; infant inability to attach on to maternal breast correctly; no observable signs of oxytocin release; observable signs of inadequate infant intake; nonsustained suckling at the breast; insufficient emptying of each breast per feeding; persistence of sore nipples beyond the first week of breastfeeding; insufficient opportunity for suckling at the breast; infant exhibiting fussiness and crying within the first hour after breastfeeding; no response to other comfort measures; infant arching and crying at the breast; resisting latching on; infant weight loss.

Related/Contributing Factors*

Prematurity; infant anomaly; maternal breast anomaly; previous breast surgery; previous history of breastfeeding failure; infant receiving supplemental feedings with artificial nipple; poor infant sucking reflex; nonsupportive partner/family; knowledge deficit; interruption in breastfeeding; maternal anxiety or ambivalence; inadequate maternal diet.

Breathing Pattern, Ineffective

(see also *Activity Intolerance; Airway Clearance, Ineffective; Gas Exchange, Impaired*)

The state in which an individual's inhalation and/or exhalation pattern does not enable adequate pulmonary inflation or emptying.

Major Defining Characteristics

Dyspnea; shortness of breath; tachypnea; fremitus; abnormal arterial blood gas; cyanosis; cough; nasal flaring; respiratory depth changes; assumption of 3-point position; pursed-lip breathing/prolonged expiratory phase; increased anteroposterior diameter; use of accessory muscles; altered chest excursion.

*Adapted by author.
§Added to the list by the author.

Related/Contributing Factors*

Neuromuscular impairment; *Pain;* musculoskeletal impairment; perception/cognitive impairment; *Anxiety; Fear;* decreased energy/fatigue; *Knowledge Deficit: Effective Breathing Patterns.*

Cardiac Output, Decreased

(see also *Activity Intolerance*)

A state in which the blood pumped by an individual's heart is sufficiently reduced that it is inadequate to meet the needs of the body's tissues.

Major Defining Characteristics

Variations in blood pressure readings; arrhythmias; fatigue; jugular vein distention; color changes, skin and mucous membranes; oliguria; decreased peripheral pulses; cold clammy skin; rales; dyspnea, orthopnea; restlessness.

Minor Defining Characteristics

Change in mental status; shortness of breath; syncope; vertigo; edema; cough; frothy sputum; gallop rhythm; weakness.

Related/Contributing Factors*

Dehydration; cardiac pathology (*e.g.,* left ventricular failure); medication side effects.

Communication, Impaired§

The state in which an individual experiences a decreased or absent ability to use or understand language in human interaction.

Major Defining Characteristics†

Inability to speak dominant language; difficulty speaking or verbalizing; refusal or inability to speak; stuttering; slurring; difficulty forming words or sentences; difficulty expressing thought verbally; inappropriate verbalization; dyspnea; disorientation; decreased ability to hear.

Related/Contributing Factors

Decrease in circulation to brain; physical barrier (brain tumor, tracheostomy, intubation); anatomical defect, cleft palate; psychological barriers (psychosis, lack of stimuli); cultural difference; developmental or age-related.

Communication, Impaired Verbal

See *Communication, Impaired.*

Conflict, Decisional (Specify)

(see also Anxiety; Coping, Ineffective Individual; Spiritual Distress)

The state in which the person experiences uncertainty about the course of action to be taken when choice among competing actions involves risk, loss, or challenge to personal life values.*

Major Defining Characteristics

Verbalized uncertainty about choices; verbalization of undesired consequences of alternative actions being considered; vacillation between alternative choices; delayed decision-making.

Minor Defining Characteristics

Verbalized feeling of distress while attempting a decision; self-focusing; physical signs of distress or tension (increased heart rate, increased muscle tension, restlessness, *etc.*); questioning of personal values and beliefs while attempting a decision.

Related/Contributing Factors

Unclear personal values/beliefs; perceived threat to value system; lack of experience or interference with decision-making; lack of relevant information; support system deficit; multiple or divergent sources of information.

Conflict, Parental Role

(see also Coping, Ineffective Family: Compromised; Coping, Ineffective Family: Disabled; Family Processes, Altered; Parenting, Altered)

The state in which a parent experiences role confusion and conflict in response to crisis.

Major Defining Characteristics

Parent(s) expresses concerns/feelings of inadequacy to provide for child's physical and emotional needs during hospital-

ization or in the home; demonstrated disruption in care-taking routines; parent(s) expresses concerns about changes in parental role, family functioning, family communication, family health.

Minor Defining Characteristics

Concern about perceived loss of control over decisions relating to their child; reluctance to participate in usual caretaking activities even with encouragement and support; verbalization or demonstration of feelings of guilt, anger, fear, anxiety and/or frustrations about effect of child's illness on family process.

Related/Contributing Factors

Separation from child because of chronic illness; intimidation with invasive or restrictive modalities (*e.g.,* isolation, intubation); specialized care centers, policies; home care of a child with special needs (*e.g.,* apnea monitoring, postural drainage, hyperalimentation); change in marital status; interruptions of family life due to home-care regimen (treatments, caregivers, lack of respite).

Constipation

(see also Constipation, Colonic; Constipation, Perceived)

A state in which an individual experiences a change in normal bowel habits characterized by a decrease in frequency and/or passage of hard, dry stools.

Major Defining Characteristics

Decreased activity level; frequency less than usual pattern; hard form stools; palpable mass; reported feeling of pressure in rectum; reported feeling of rectal fullness; straining at stool.

Minor Defining Characteristics

Abdominal pain; appetite impairment; back pain; headache; interference with daily living; use of laxatives.

Related/Contributing Factors*

Bedrest; diet deficient in fluids and/or roughage; lack of exercise; side effects of medications.

Constipation, Colonic

(see also Constipation; Constipation, Perceived)

The state in which an individual's pattern of elimination is characterized by hard, dry stool that results from a delay in passage of food residue.

*Adapted by author.

Major Defining Characteristics

Decreased frequency; hard, dry stool; straining at stool; painful defecation; abdominal distention; palpable mass.

Minor Defining Characteristics

Rectal pressure; headache; appetite impairment; abdominal pain.

Related/Contributing Factors

Less than adequate fluid intake; less than adequate dietary intake; less than adequate fiber; less than adequate physical activity; immobility; lack of privacy; emotional disturbances; chronic use of medication and enemas; stress; change in daily routine; metabolic problems, *e.g.*, hypothyroidism, hypocalcemia, hypokalemia.

Constipation, Perceived

(see also *Constipation; Constipation, Colonic*)

The state in which an individual makes a self-diagnosis of constipation and ensures a daily bowel movement through abuse of laxatives, enemas, and suppositories.

Major Defining Characteristics

Expectation of a daily bowel movement with the resulting overuse of laxatives, enemas, and suppositories; expected passage of stool at same time every day.

Related/Contributing Factors

Cultural/family health beliefs; faulty appraisal; impaired thought processes.

Coping, Defensive

(see also *Coping, Ineffective Individual*)

The state in which an individual repeatedly projects falsely positive self-evaluation based on a self-protective pattern that defends against underlying perceived threats to positive self-regard.

Major Defining Characteristics

Denial of obvious problems/weaknesses; projection of blame/responsibility; rationalization failures; hypersensitivity to slight/criticism; grandiosity.

*Adapted by author.

Minor Defining Characteristics

Superior attitude toward others; difficulty establishing/maintaining relationships; hostile laughter or ridicule of others; difficulty in reality testing perceptions; lack of follow-through or participation in treatment or therapy.

Related/Contributing Factors*

Anxiety; fear.

Coping, Family: Potential for Growth

Effective management of adaptive tasks by family member involved with the client's health challenge, who now is exhibiting desire and readiness for enhanced health and growth in regard to self and in relation to the client.

Major Defining Characteristics

Family member attempting to describe growth impact of crisis on his or her own values, priorities, goal, or relationships; family member moving in direction of health-promoting and enriching life-style that supports and monitors maturational processes, audits and negotiates treatment programs, and generally chooses experiences that optimize wellness; individual expressing interest in making contact on a one-to-one basis or on a mutual-aid group basis with another person who has experienced a similar situation.

Related/Contributing Factors*

Needs sufficiently gratified and adaptive tasks effectively addressed to enable goals of self-actualization to surface; knowledge of personal and community resources.

Coping, Ineffective Family: Compromised

(see also *Coping, Ineffective Family: Disabling; Family Processes, Altered; Parenting, Altered*)

The state in which family members experience insufficient or ineffective support (usually by a primary person, such as a family member or close friend) to adapt to a life challenge (*e.g.*, chronic illness, loss).*

Major Defining Characteristics

Subjective: client expresses or confirms a concern or complaint about significant other's response to his or with personal reactions (*e.g.*, fear, anticipatory grief, guilt, anxiety, to client's illness or disability or to other situational or developmental crises); significant person describes or confirms inadequate understanding or knowledge base that interferes with effective assistive or supportive behaviors.

Objective: significant person attempts assistive or supportive behaviors with less than satisfactory results; significant person withdraws or enters into limited or temporary personal communication with the client at the time of need; significant person displays protective behavior disproportionate (too little or too much) to the client's abilities or need for autonomy.

Related/Contributing Factors

Inadequate or incorrect information or understanding by a primary person; temporary preoccupation by a significant person who is trying to manage emotional conflicts and personal suffering and is unable to perceive or act effectively in regard to client's needs; temporary family disorganization and role changes; other situational or developmental crises or situations the significant person may be facing; little support provided by client, in turn, for primary person; prolonged disease or disability progression that exhausts supportive capacity of significant people.

Coping, Ineffective Family: Disabling
(see also *Coping, Ineffective Family: Compromised; Parenting, Altered; Family Processes, Altered; Conflict, Parental Role*)

Behavior of a significant person (family member or other primary person) that disables his or her own capacities and the client's capacities to effectively address tasks essential to either person's adaptation to the health challenge.

Major Defining Characteristics

Neglectful care of the client in regard to basic human needs and/or illness treatment; distortion of reality regarding the client's health problem, including extreme denial about its existence or severity; intolerance; rejection; abandonment; desertion; carrying on usual routines, disregarding client's needs; psychosomaticism; taking on illness signs of client; decisions and actions by family that are detrimental to economic or social well-being; agitation, depression, aggression, hostility; impaired restructuring of a meaningful life for self, impaired individualization, prolonged over-concern for client; neglectful relationships with other family members; client's development of helpless, inactive dependence.

*Adapted by author.

Related/Contributing Factors

Significant person with chronically unexpressed feelings of guilt, anxiety, hostility, despair, *etc.;* dissonant discrepancy of coping styles for dealing with adaptive tasks by the significant person and client or among significant people; highly ambivalent family relationships; arbitrary handling of family's resistance to treatment, which tends to solidify defensiveness as it fails to deal adequately with underlying anxiety.

Coping, Ineffective Individual

Impairment of adaptive behaviors and problem-solving abilities of a person in meeting life's demands and roles.

Major Defining Characteristics

Verbalization of inability to cope or inability to ask for help; inability to meet role expectations; inability to meet basic needs; inability to problem-solve; alteration in societal participation; destructive behavior toward self or others; inappropriate use of defense mechanisms; change in usual communication patterns; verbal manipulation; high illness rate; high rate of accidents.

Related/Contributing Factors*

Situational crises; maturational crises; personal vulnerability; fear; lack of knowledge of personal and community resources.

Denial, Ineffective
(see also *Coping, Ineffective Individual*)

The state of a conscious or unconscious attempt to disavow the knowledge or meaning of an event to reduce anxiety/fear to the detriment of health.

Major Defining Characteristics

Delay of seeking or refusal of healthcare attention to the detriment of health; lack of perception of personal relevance of symptoms or danger.

Minor Defining Characteristics

Use of home remedies (self-treatment) to relieve symptoms; denial of fear of death or invalidism; minimalization of symptoms; displacement of source of symptoms to other organs; inability to admit impact of disease on life pattern; dismissive gestures or comments when speaking of distressing events; displacement of fear of impact of the condition; display of inappropriate affect.

Related/Contributing Factors*

Fear; alcohol abuse; drug abuse; type "A" personality.

Diarrhea
(see also *Bowel Incontinence*)

A state in which an individual experiences a change in normal bowel habits characterized by the frequent passage of loose, fluid, unformed stools.

Major Defining Characteristics

Abdominal pain; cramping; increased frequency; increased frequency of bowel sounds; loose liquid stools; urgency.

Minor Defining Characteristics

Change in color.

Related/Contributing Factors*

Side effects of medications; tube feedings; laxative abuse; anxiety.

Disuse, Potential for

A state in which an individual is at risk for deterioration of body systems as the result of prescribed or unavoidable musculoskeletal inactivity.

Defining Characteristics

Presence of risk factors such as paralysis; mechanical immobilization; prescribed immobilization; severe pain; altered level of consciousness.

Diversional Activity Deficit

The state in which an individual experiences a decreased stimulation from or interest or engagement in recreational or leisure activities.

Major Defining Characteristics

Patient's statements regarding boredom, wish there were something to do, read, *etc.*; usual hobbies cannot be undertaken in hospital; failure to thrive.*

*Adapted by author.

Related/Contributing Factors*

Environmental lack of diversional activity, *e.g.,* long-term hospitalization, frequent lengthy treatments; extremes of age (very young and elderly); developmental delay; deafness; blindness; chronic fatigue; chronic pain; lack of knowledge of personal and community resources.

Dysreflexia

The state in which an individual with a spinal cord injury at T7 or above experiences a life threatening, uninhibited, sympathetic response of the nervous system to a noxious stimulus.

Major Defining Characteristics

Individual with spinal cord injury (T7 or above) with paroxysmal hypertension (sudden periodic elevated blood pressure where systolic pressure is over 140 mmHg and diastolic is above 90 mmHg); bradycardia or tachycardia (pulse rate of less than 60 or over 100 beats per minute); diaphoresis (above the injury); red splotches on skin (above the injury); pallor (below the injury); headache (a diffuse pain in different portions of the head and not confined to any nerve distribution area).

Minor Defining Characteristics

Chilling; conjunctival congestion; Horner's Syndrome (contraction of the pupil, partial ptosis of the eyelid, enophthalmos and sometimes loss of sweating over the affected side of the face); paresthesia; pilomotor reflex (gooseflesh formation when skin is cooled); blurred vision; chest pain; metallic taste in mouth; nasal congestion.

Related/Contributing Factors

Bladder distention; bowel distention; skin irritation.

Family Processes, Altered
(see also *Coping, Ineffective Family; Conflict, Parental Role; Parenting, Altered*)

The state in which a family that normally functions effectively experiences a dysfunction.

Major Defining Characteristics

Family system unable to meet physical needs of its members; family system unable to meet emotional needs of its members; family system unable to meet spiritual needs of its members; parents do not demonstrate respect for each other's views on child-rearing practices; inability to express/accept wide range of feelings; inability to express/accept feelings of members; family unable to meet security needs of its members; inability of the family members to relate to each other for mutual growth and maturation; family uninvolved in community activities; inability to accept/receive help appropriately; rigidity in function and roles; family not demonstrating respect for individuality and autonomy of its members; family unable to adapt to change/deal with traumatic experience constructively; family failing to accomplish current/past developmental task; unhealthy family decision-making process; failure to send and receive clear messages; inappropriate boundary maintenance; inappropriate/poorly communicated family rules, rituals, symbols; unexamined family myths; inappropriate level and direction of energy.

Related/Contributing Factors

Situation transition and/or crises; developmental transition and/or crisis.

Fatigue
(see also Activity Intolerance)

An overwhelming sustained sense of exhaustion and decreased capacity for physical and mental work.

Major Defining Characteristics

Verbalization of an unremitting and overwhelming lack of energy; inability to maintain usual routines.

Minor Defining Characteristics

Perceived need for additional energy to accomplish routine tasks; increase in physical complaints; emotionally labile or irritable; impaired ability to concentrate; decreased performance; lethargy or listlessness; disinterest in surroundings/introspection; decreased libido; accident prone.

Related/Contributing Factors

Decreased/increased metabolic energy production; overwhelming psychological or emotional demands; increased energy requirements to perform activity of daily living; excessive social and/or role demands; states of discomfort; altered body chemistry (e.g., medications, drug withdrawal, chemotherapy).

Fear
(see also Anxiety)

Feeling of dread related to an identifiable source that the person validates.

*Adapted by author.

Major Defining Characteristic

Ability to identify object of fear.

Related/Contributing Factors*

Previous experience with similar situation; lack of presence of significant other, communication barrier.

Fluid Volume Deficit, Actual*
(see also Fluid Volume Deficit, Potential)

The state in which an individual experiences vascular, cellular, or intracellular dehydration.

Major Defining Characteristic*

Increased serum sodium levels.*

Minor Defining Characteristics*

Poor skin turgor, or interstial edema with dry mouth/thirst; increased pulse rate; decreased pulse volume/pressure; increased body temperature; dry skin; hemoconcentration; weakness.

Related/Contributing Factors*

Organ or system disease; organ immaturity; decreased fluid intake; increased salt intake; deconditioned state; extremes of age; extremes of weight; excessive losses through normal routes (e.g., diarrhea); loss of fluid through abnormal routes (e.g., indwelling tubes); deviations affecting access to or intake or absorption of fluids (e.g., physical immobility); factors influencing fluid needs (e.g, hypermetabolic states); knowledge deficit of fluid needs; medications (e.g., diuretics) depression; excessive heat.

Fluid Volume Deficit, Potential
(see also Fluid Volume Deficit, Actual)

The state in which an individual is at risk of experiencing vascular, cellular, or intracellular dehydration.

Major Defining Characteristics

Increased output; urinary frequency; thirst; altered intake; fever.

Related/Contributing Factors*

Same as Fluid Volume Deficit, Actual.

Fluid Volume Excess

(see also *Cardiac Output, Decreased*)

The state in which an individual experiences increased fluid retention and edema.

Major Defining Characteristics

Edema; effusion; anasarca; weight gain; shortness of breath, orthopnea; intake greater than output; S/3 heart sound; pulmonary congestion (chest x-ray); abnormal breath sounds, rales (crackles); change in respiratory pattern; change in mental status; decreased hemoglobin and hematocrit; blood pressure changes; central venous pressure changes; pulmonary artery pressure changes; jugular vein distention; positive hepatojugular reflex; oliguria; specific gravity changes; azotemia; altered electrolytes; restlessness and anxiety.

Related/Contributing Factors

Organ or system disease or immaturity; excess fluid intake; excess sodium intake.

Gas Exchange, Impaired

(see also *Activity Intolerance; Breathing Pattern, Ineffective*)

The state in which the individual experiences a decreased passage of oxygen and/or carbon dioxide between the alveoli of the lungs and the vascular system.

Major Defining Characteristics

Confusion; somnolence; restlessness; irritability; inability to move secretions; hypercapnea; hypoxia; abnormal pulse rate.

Related/Contributing Factors*

Ventilation perfusion imbalance; organ or system disease or immaturity.

Grieving§

That state in which an individual or family experiences extreme feelings of sadness related to an actual or perceived loss (of object, loved one, or normal capabilities).*

*Adapted by author.
§Added to the list by the author.

Major Defining Characteristics*

Verbal expression of distress at loss; denial of loss; expression of guilt; expression of unresolved issues; anger; sadness; crying; difficulty in expressing loss; alterations in eating habits, sleep patterns, dream patterns, activity level, libido; idealization of lost object; reliving of past experiences; interference with life functioning; developmental regression; labile affect; alterations in concentration and/or pursuits of tasks.

Related/Contributing Factors*

Actual or perceived object loss (object loss is used in the broadest sense and may include people, possessions, a job, status, home, ideals, parts and processes of the body).

Grieving, Anticipatory

The state in which an individual or family experiences feelings of anxiety, fear, or sadness related to a possible loss (of object, loved one, or normal capabilities).*

Major Defining Characteristics

Potential loss of significant object; expression of distress at potential loss; denial of potential loss; guilt; anger; sorrow; chokes feelings; change in eating habits; alterations in sleep patterns; alterations in activity level; altered libido; altered communication patterns.

Related/Contributing Factors

Anticipated object loss (object loss is used in the broadest sense, and may include people, possessions, a job, status, home, ideals, parts and processes of the body).

Grieving, Dysfunctional
See *Grieving*.

Growth and Development, Altered

The state in which an individual demonstrates deviations in norms from his or her age group.

Major Defining Characteristics

Delay or difficulty in performing skills (motor, social, or expressive) typical of age group; altered physical growth; inability to perform self-care or self-control activities appropriate for age.

Minor Defining Characteristics

Flat affect; listlessness, decreased responses.

Related/Contributing Factors

Inadequate caretaking; indifference, inconsistent responsiveness, multiple caretakers; separation from significant others; environmental and stimulation deficiencies; effects of physical disability; prescribed dependence.

Health Maintenance, Altered

Inability to identify, manage, and/or seek out help to maintain health.

Major Defining Characteristics

Demonstrated lack of knowledge regarding basic health practices; demonstrated lack of adaptive behaviors to internal/external environmental changes; reported or observed inability to take responsibility for meeting basic health practices in any or all functional pattern areas; history of lack of *Health Seeking Behavior;* expressed interest in improving health behaviors; reported or observed lack of equipment, financial and/or other resources; reported or observed impairment of personal support systems.

Related/Contributing Factors

Lack of or significant alterations in communication skills (written, verbal and/or gestural); lack of ability to make deliberate and thoughtful judgments; perceptual/cognitive impairment (complete/partial lack of gross and/or fine motor skills); *Ineffective Individual Coping; Dysfunctional Grieving;* unachieved developmental tasks; ineffective family coping; disabling spiritual distress; lack of material resources.

Health Seeking Behavior (Specify)

A state in which an individual in stable health is actively seeking ways to alter personal health habits, and/or the environment in order to move toward a higher level of health.*

Major Defining Characteristic

Expressed or observed desire to seek a higher level of wellness.

*Adapted by author.

Minor Defining Characteristics

Expressed or observed desire for increased control of health practice; expression of concern about current environmental conditions on health status; stated or observed unfamiliarity with wellness community resources; demonstrated or observed lack of knowledge in health promotion behaviors.

Home Maintenance Management, Impaired
(see also *Injury, Potential for*)

Inability to independently maintain a safe, growth-promoting, immediate environment.

Major Defining Characteristics*

Subjective: household members express difficulty in maintaining their home in a comfortable fashion; household requests assistance with home maintenance; household members describe outstanding debts or financial crises.

Objective: disorderly surroundings; unwashed or unavailable cooking equipment, clothes, or linen; accumulation of dirt, food wastes, or hygienic wastes; offensive odors; inappropriate household temperature; overtaxed family members (*e.g.,* exhausted, anxious); lack of necessary equipment or aids; presence of vermin or rodents; repeated hygienic disorders, infestations, or infections; evidence of hazards in the home.

Related/Contributing Factors*

Individual/family member disease or injury; insufficient family organization or planning; insufficient finances; unfamiliarity with neighborhood resources; impaired cognitive or emotional functioning; lack of knowledge; lack of role modeling; inadequate support systems; young children in home.

Hopelessness
(see also *Powerlessness*)

A state in which an individual sees limited or no alternatives or personal choices available and is unable to mobilize energy on his or her own behalf.

Major Defining Characteristics

Passivity, decreased verbalization; decreased affect; verbal cues (despondent content, "I can't," sighing).

Minor Defining Characteristics*

Lack of initiative; decreased response to stimuli; decreased affect; turning away from speaker; closing eyes; shrugging in response to speaker; decreased appetite; increased sleep; lack of involvement in care/passively allowing care; verbalizations of anger.

Related/Contributing Factors*

Prolonged activity restriction creating isolation; failing or deteriorating physiological condition; long-term stress; abandonment; lost belief in transcendent values/God; unavailable financial/personal resources.

Hyperthermia

[Note: Hyperthermia is also a medical diagnosis (see Tabor's Medical Dictionary.]

A state in which an individual's body temperature is elevated above his or her normal range.

Major Defining Characteristics

Increase in body temperature above normal range.

Minor Defining Characteristics

Flushed skin; warm to touch; increased respiratory rate; tachycardia; seizures/convulsions.

Related/Contributing Factors

Exposure to hot environment; vigorous activity; medications/anesthesia; inappropriate clothing; increased metabolic rate; illness or trauma; dehydration; inability or decreased ability to perspire.

Hypothermia

[Note: Author recommends this diagnosis be used as a potential diagnosis only. Actual hypothermia (i.e., temperature below 95°F) should be referred to the physician.]

The state in which an individual's body temperature is reduced below 95°F.*

Major Defining Characteristics*

Reduction in body temperature below normal range; shivering (mild); cool skin; pallor (moderate).

Minor Defining Characteristics

Confusion; slow capillary refill; tachycardia; cyanotic nail beds; hypertension; piloerection.

Related/Contributing Factors*

Exposure to cool or cold environment; illness or trauma; damage to hypothalamus; inability or decreased ability to shiver; malnutrition; inadequate clothing; consumption of alcohol; medications causing vasodilation; evaporation of moisture from skin in cool environment; decreased metabolic rate, inactivity; aging; neonatal period; prematurity.

Infection, Potential for

The state in which an individual is at increased risk for being invaded by pathogenic organisms.

Defining Characteristics/Risk Factors*

Inadequate primary defenses (broken skin, traumatized tissue, decreased, ciliary action, stasis of body fluids, change in pH of secretions, altered peristalsis); inadequate secondary defenses (decreased hemoglobin, leukopenia, immunosuppression; inadequate acquired immunity; chronic disease; malnutrition); environmental hazards (work, travel); treatment-related hazards (invasive lines/procedures, childbirth, medications); *Knowledge Deficit: Self-protection;* extremes of age.

Injury, Potential for

(see also Poisoning, Potential for; Suffocating, Potential for; Trauma, Potential for; Home Maintenance Management, Impaired)

The state in which the individual is at risk for injury as a result of the presence of individual risk factors or environmental hazards.*

Major Defining Characteristics/Risk Factors*

History of frequent injury/accidents; presence of individual risk factors (e.g., extremes of age, deconditioned state, difficulty ambulating, lack of knowledge of hazards); presence of environmental risk factors (e.g., steps in poor repair, poor lighting, lack of handrails or siderails).

Knowledge Deficit (Specify)

The state in which the individual lacks the skills or information to successfully manage his/her own healthcare.*

*Adapted by author.

Major Defining Characteristics

Verbalization of the problem; inaccurate follow-through of instruction; inaccurate performance of test; inappropriate or exaggerated behaviors (*e.g.,* hysteria, hostility, agitation, apathy).

Related/Contributing Factors*

Lack of exposure; lack of recall; information misinterpretation; cognitive limitation; lack of interest in learning (no motivation); unfamiliarity with information resources; *Fear; Denial;* lack of accessible written information to reinforce learning.*

Mobility, Impaired Physical

A state in which the individual experiences a limitation of ability for independent physical movement.

Major Defining Characteristics

Inability to purposefully move within the physical environment, including bed mobility, transfer, and ambulation; reluctance to attempt movement; limited range of motion; decreased muscle strength, control and/or mass; imposed restrictions of movement, including mechanical, medical protocol; impaired coordination.

Related/Contributing Factors

Intolerance to activity/decreased strength and endurance; pain/discomfort; perceptual/cognitive impairment; neuromuscular impairment; musculoskeletal impairment; depression/severe anxiety.

Suggested Code for Functional Level Classification

0 = Completely independent.

1 = Requires use of equipment or device.

2 = Requires help from another person, for assistance, supervision, or teaching.

3 = Requires help from another person and equipment device.

4 = Dependent, does not participate in activity.

*Adapted by author.

Noncompliance

The state in which the individual expresses a desire to conform with therapeutic regimen, but is unable to demonstrate observable signs of following the regimen.*

Major Defining Characteristics*

Statements of having difficulty with therapeutic regimen; lack of knowledge of therapeutic regimen; lack of available personal and community resources.

Related/Contributing Factors*

Complicated or prolonged regimen.

Nutrition, Altered: Less Than Body Requirements

The state in which an individual experiences an intake of nutrients insufficient to meet metabolic needs.

Major Defining Characteristics

Loss of weight with adequate food intake; body weight 20% or more under ideal; reported inadequate food intake less than RDA (recommended daily allowance); weakness of muscles required for swallowing or mastication; reported or evidence of lack of food; aversion to eating; reported altered taste sensation; satiety immediately after ingesting food; abdominal pain with or without pathology; sore, inflamed buccal cavity; capillary fragility; abdominal cramping; diarrhea and/or steatorrhea; hyperactive bowel sounds; lack of interest in food; perceived inability to ingest food; pale conjunctival and mucous membranes; poor muscle tone; excessive loss of hair; lack of information, misinformation; misconceptions.

Related/Contributing Factors

Inability to ingest or digest food or absorb nutrients because of biological, psychological, or economic factors.

Nutrition, Altered: More Than Body Requirements

[Note: Also listed as a potential diagnosis.]

The state in which an individual is experiencing an intake of nutrients that exceeds metabolic needs.

Major Defining Characteristics

Weight 10%–20% over ideal for height and frame; triceps skin fold greater than 15 mm in men, 25 mm in women; sedentary

sedentary activity level; reported or observed dysfunctional eating patterns; pairing food with other activities; concentrating food intake at end of day; eating in response to external cues such as time of day, social situation; eating in response to internal cues other than hunger (e.g., Anxiety).*

Related/Contributing Factors*

Excessive intake in relation to metabolic need; poor dietary habits; sedentary lifestyle; ineffective coping: pregnancy; lack of knowledge of nutritional value of foods.

Nutrition, Altered: Potential For More Than Body Requirements

The state in which an individual is at risk of experiencing an intake of nutrients which exceeds metabolic needs.

Major Defining Characteristics

Reported or observed obesity in one or both parents; rapid transition across growth percentiles in infants or children; reported use of solid food as major food source before 5 months of age; observed use of food as reward or comfort measure; reported or observed higher baseline weight at beginning of each pregnancy; dysfunctional eating patterns: pairing food with other activities; concentrating food intake at end of day; eating in response to external cues such as time of day, social situation; eating in response to internal cues other than hunger such as Anxiety.

Related Factors

Hereditary predisposition; excessive intake during late gestational life, early infancy, and adolescence; frequent closely spaced pregnancies; dysfunctional psychological conditioning in relation to food; membership in lower socioeconomic group.

Oral Mucous Membrane, Altered

The state in which an individual experiences disruptions in the tissue layers of the oral cavity.

Major Defining Characteristics

Oral pain/discomfort; coated tongue; xerostomia (dry mouth); stomatitis; oral lesions or ulcers; lack of or decreased sali-

vation; leukoplakia; edema; hyperemia; oral plaque; desquamation; vesicles; hemorrhagic gingivitis, carious teeth; halitosis.

Related/Contributing Factors*

Pathological conditions—oral cavity (radiation to head or neck); dehydration; trauma (chemical, mechanical); NPO for more than 24 hours; ineffective oral hygiene; mouth breathing; malnutrition; infection; lack of or decreased salivation; medication.

Pain
(see also Pain, Chronic)

A state in which an individual experiences and reports the presence of severe discomfort or an uncomfortable sensation.

Major Defining Characteristics

Subjective: communication (verbal or coded) of pain descriptors.

Objective: guarded or protective behavior; self-focusing; narrowed focus (altered time perception, withdrawal from social contact, impaired thought process); distraction behavior (moaning, crying, pacing, seeking out other people and/or activities, restlessness); facial mask of pain (eyes lackluster, "beaten look," fixed or scattered movement, grimace); alteration in muscle tone (may span from listness to rigid); autonomic responses not seen in chronic stable pain (diaphoresis, blood pressure and pulse change, pupillary dilation, increased or decreased respiratory rate).

Related/Contributing Factors*

Injuring agents (biological, chemical, physical, psychological); organ or system disease; drug tolerance/addiction.

Pain, Chronic
(see also Pain)

A state in which the individual experiences pain that continues for more than six months in duration.

Major Defining Characteristics

Verbal report or observed evidence of pain experienced for more than 6 months.

*Adapted by author.

Minor Defining Characteristics

Fear of re-injury; physical and social withdrawal; altered ability to continue previous activities; anorexia; weight changes; changes in sleep patterns; facial mask; guarded movement.

Related/Contributing Factors*

Chronic physical/psychosocial disability; depression, organ or system disease; drug tolerance/addiction.

Parenting, Altered

[Note: It is important to state as a preface to this diagnosis that adjustment to parenting in general is a normal maturational process that elicits nursing behaviors of prevention of potential problems and health promotion.]

The ability of nuturing figure(s) to create an environment that promotes the optimum growth and development of another human being.

Major Defining Characteristics

Abandonment; runaway; verbalization, cannot control child; incidence of physical and psychological trauma; lack of parental attachment behaviors; inappropriate visual, tactile, auditory stimulation; negative identification of infant/child's characteristics; negative attachment of meanings to infant/child's characteristics; constant verbalization of disappointment in gender or physical characteristics of the infant/child; verbalization of resentment toward the infant/child; verbalization of role inadequacy; inattentive to infant/child's needs; verbal disgust at body functions of infant/child; noncompliance with health appointments for self and/or infant/child; inappropriate caretaking behaviors (toilet training, sleep/rest, feeding); inappropriate or inconsistent discipline practices; frequent accidents; frequent illness; growth and development lag in the child; history of child abuse or abandonment by primary caretaker; verbalizes desire to have child call him/herself by first name vs. traditional cultural tendencies; child receives care from multiple caretakers without consideration for the needs of the infant/child; compulsive search for role approval from others.

Related Factors

Lack of available role model; ineffective role model; physical and psychosocial abuse of nurturing figure; lack of support between/from significant other(s); unmet social/emotional maturation needs of parenting figures; interruption in bonding

*Adapted by author.

process, i.e., maternal, paternal, other; unrealistic expectation for self, infant, partner; perceived threat to own survival, physical and emotional; mental and/or physical illness; presence of stress (financial, legal, recent crisis, cultural move); lack of knowledge; limited cognitive functioning; lack of role identity; lack of inappropriate response of child to relationship; multiple pregnancies.

Parenting, Potential Altered
(see also Coping, Ineffective Family: Compromised; Coping, Ineffective Family: Disabled; Family Processes, Altered; Conflict, Parental Role)

The state in which a nurturing figure(s) of a family is at risk for inability to provide an environment that promotes optimum growth and development of another human being.*

Major Defining Characteristics

Lack of parental attachment behaviors; inappropriate visual, tactile, auditory stimulation of child; negative identification of infant/child's characteristics; negative attachment of meanings to infant/child's characteristics; constant verbalization of disappointment in gender or physical characteristics of the infant/child; verbalization of resentment towards the infant/child; verbalization of role inadequacy; lack of attention to infant/child's needs; verbal disgust at body functions of infant/child; noncompliance with health appointments for self and/or infant/child; inappropriate caretaking behaviors (toilet training, sleep/rest, feeding); inappropriate or inconsistent discipline practices; frequent accidents; frequent illness; growth and development lag in the child; history of child abuse or abandonment by primary caretaker; verbalized desire to have child call him/herself by first name vs. traditional cultural tendencies; child receives care from multiple caretakers without consideration for the needs of the infant/child; compulsive search for role approval from others.

Related/Contributing Factors

Lack of available role model; ineffective role model; physical and psychosocial abuse of nurturing figure; lack of support between/from significant other(s); unmet social/emotional maturation needs of parenting figures; interruption in bonding process (maternal, paternal, other); unrealistic expectation for self, infant, partner; perceived threat to own survival, physical and emotional; mental and/or physical illness; presence of stress (financial, legal, recent crisis, cultural move); lack of knowledge; limited cognitive functioning; lack of role identity; lack of inappropriate response of child to relationship; multiple pregnancies.

Personal Identity Disturbance

The inability to distinguish between self and nonself.

[Note: Major Defining Characteristics and Related/Contributing Factors have not been developed by NANDA. Added by author.]

Major Defining Characteristics

Verbalization of being someone/something other than self.

Related/Contributing Factor

Mental illness.

Poisoning, Potential for
(see also *Home Maintenance Management, Impaired*)

Accentuated risk of accidental exposure to or ingestion of drugs or dangerous products in doses sufficient to cause poisoning.

Major Defining Characteristics/Risk Factors

Individual: reduced vision; verbalization of occupational setting without adequate safeguards; lack of safety or drug education; lack of proper precaution; cognitive or emotional difficulties; insufficient finances.

Environmental: large supplies of drugs in house; medicines stored in unlocked cabinets accessible to children or confused persons; dangerous products placed or stored within the reach of children or confused persons; availability of illicit drugs potentially contaminated by poisonous additives; flaking, peeling paint, or plaster in presence of young children; chemical contamination of food and water; unprotected contact with heavy metals or chemicals; paint, lacquer, *etc.,* in poorly ventilated areas or without effective protection; presence of poisonous vegetation; presence of atmospheric pollutants.

Post-Trauma Response

The state of an individual experiencing a sustained painful response to an unexpected extraordinary life event(s).

*Adapted by author.

Major Defining Characteristics

Re-experience of the traumatic event that may be identified in cognitive, affective, and/or sensory motor activities (flashbacks, intrusive thoughts, repetitive dreams or nightmares, excessive verbalization of the traumatic event, verbalization of survival guilt or guilt about behavior required for survival).

Minor Defining Characteristics

Psychic/emotional numbness (impaired interpretation of reality, confusion, dissociation or amnesia, vagueness about traumatic event, constricted affect); altered lifestyle (self-destructiveness, such as substance abuse, suicide attempt or other acting out behavior, difficulty with interpersonal relationships, development of phobia regarding trauma, poor impulse control/irritability and explosiveness).

Related/Contributing Factors

Disasters, wars; epidemics; rape; assault; torture; catastrophic illness or accident.

Powerlessness
(see also *Hopelessness*)

The perception that one's own action will not significantly affect an outcome; a perceived lack of control over a current situation or immediate happening.

Major Defining Characteristics

Severe: verbal expressions of having no control or influence over a situation; verbal expressions of having no control or influence over outcome; verbal expressions of having no control over self-care; depression over physical deterioration that occurs despite patient compliance with regimens; apathy.

Moderate: nonparticipation in care or decision-making when opportunities are provided; expressions of dissatisfaction and frustration over inability to perform previous tasks and/or activities; does not monitor progress; expression of doubt regarding role performance; reluctance to express true feelings, fearing alienation from care-givers; passivity; inability to seek information regarding care; dependence on others that may result in irritability, resentment, anger, and guilt; lack of defense of self-care practices when challenged.

Low: expressions of uncertainty about fluctuating energy levels; passivity.

Related/Contributing Factors

Healthcare environment; interpersonal interactions; illness-related regimen; lifestyle of helplessness.

Rape-Trauma Syndrome

(see also *Rape Trauma Syndrome: Compound Reaction; Rape Trauma Syndrome: Silent Reaction*)

Forced, violent sexual penetration against the victim's will and consent. The trauma syndrome that develops from this attack or attempted attack includes an acute phase of disorganization of the victim's lifestyle and a long-term process of reorganization of lifestyle.

Major Defining Characteristics

Acute phase: emotional reactions (anger, embarrassment, fear of physical violence and death, humiliation, revenge, self-blame); multiple physical symptoms (gastrointestinal irritability, genitourinary discomfort, muscle tension, sleep pattern disturbance).

Long-term phase: changes in lifestyle (changes in residence; dealing with repetitive nightmares and phobias; seeking family support; seeking social network support).

Related/Contributing Factor*

Any type of sexual abuse.

Rape-Trauma Syndrome: Compound Reaction

(see also *Rape-Trauma Syndrome; Rape-Trauma Syndrome: Silent Reaction*)

The forced, violent, sexual penetration against the victim's will and consent. The trauma syndrome that develops from this attack or attempted attack includes an acute phase of disorganization of the victim's lifestyle and a long-term process of reorganization of lifestyle.

Major Defining Characteristics

Acute phase: emotional reactions (anger, embarrassment, fear of physical violence and death, humiliation, revenge, self-blame); multiple physical symptoms (gastrointestinal irritability, genitourinary discomfort, muscle tension, sleep pattern disturbance); reactivated symptoms of such previous conditions, *i.e.,* physical illness, psychiatric illness; reliance on alcohol and/or drugs.

Long-term phase: changes in lifestyle (changes in residence, repetitive nightmares and phobias, search for family support, search for social network support).

*Adapted by author.

Rape-Trauma Syndrome: Silent Reaction

(see also *Rape-Trauma Syndrome; Rape-Trauma Syndrome: Compound Reaction*)

The forced, violent sexual penetration against the victim's will and consent. The trauma syndrome that develops from this attack or attempted attack includes an acute phase of disorganization of the victim's lifestyle and a long-term process of reorganization of lifestyle.

Major Defining Characteristic

Abrupt changes in relationships with men; increase in nightmares; increased anxiety during interview (*i.e.,* blocking of associations, long periods of silence, minor stuttering, physical distress); pronounced changes in sexual behavior; no verbalization of the occurrence of rape; sudden onset of phobic reactions.

Role Performance, Altered

The state in which the individual has difficulty establishing positive relationships (*e.g.,* sexual, parental, work).*

Major Defining Characteristic

Self-verbalization of dissatisfaction with role performance.

Minor Defining Characteristics

Verbalization of dissatisfaction with role performance by others.

Self-Care Deficit, Bathing/Hygiene

A state in which the individual experiences an impaired ability to perform or complete bathing/hygiene activities for oneself.

Major Defining Characteristics

Inability to wash body or body parts; inability to obtain or get to water source; inability to regulate temperature or flow.

Related/Contributing Factors

Intolerance to activity, decreased strength and endurance; pain, discomfort; perceptual or cognitive impairment; neuromuscular impairment; depression, severe anxiety.

Self-Care Deficit, Dressing/Grooming

A state in which the individual experiences an impaired ability to perform or complete dressing and grooming activities for oneself.

Major Defining Characteristics

Impaired ability to put on or take off necessary items of clothing; impaired ability to obtain or replace articles of clothing; impaired ability to fasten clothing; inability to maintain appearance at a satisfactory level.

Related/Contributing Factors

Intolerance to activity, decreased strength and endurance; pain, discomfort; perceptual or cognitive impairment; neuromuscular impairment; musculoskeletal impairment; depression, severe anxiety.

Self-Care Deficit, Feeding

A state in which the individual experiences an impaired ability to perform or complete feeding activities for oneself.

Major Defining Characteristics

Inability to bring food from a receptacle to the mouth.

Related/Contributing Factors

Intolerance to activity, decreased strength and endurance; pain, discomfort; perceptual or cognitive impairment; neuromuscular impairment; musculoskeletal impairment; depression, severe anxiety.

Self-Care Deficit, Toileting

A state in which the individual experiences an impaired ability to perform or complete toileting activities for oneself.

Major Defining Characteristics

Inability to get to toilet; inability to sit on or rise from toilet; inability to manipulate clothing for toileting; inability to carry out proper toilet hygiene; inability to flush toilet or commode.

*Adapted by author.

Related/Contributing Factors

Impaired transfer ability; impaired mobility status; intolerance to activity, decreased strength and endurance; pain, discomfort; perceptual or cognitive impairment; neuromuscular impairment; musculoskeletal impairment; depression, severe anxiety.

Self-Esteem Disturbance
(see also *Self-Esteem, Situational Low; Self-Esteem, Chronic Low*)

A disruption in the way one perceives one's self-esteem.

Major Defining Characteristics/Related Factors*

Verbalization of feeling different about oneself than usual; (may be self-deprecating or grandiose); history of abuse (verbal, sexual, physical), illness, disability.

Self-Esteem, Chronic Low

Long standing negative self-evaluation/feelings about self or self capabilities.

Major Defining Characteristics

Long standing or chronic; self-negating verbalization; expressions of shame/guilt; evaluates self as unable to deal with events; rationalizes away/rejects positive feedback and exaggerates; negative feedback about self; hesitant to try new things/situations.

Minor Defining Characteristics

Frequent lack of success in work or other life events; overly conforming; dependent on others' opinions; lack of eye contact; nonassertive/passive; indecisive; excessively seeks reassurance.

Self-Esteem, Situational Low
(see also *Self-Esteem, Chronic Low; Self-Esteem Disturbance*)

The negative self-evaluation and feelings about the self that develop in response to a loss or change in an individual who previously had a positive self-evaluation.

Major Defining Characteristics

Episodic occurrence of negative self-appraisal in response to life events in a person with a previous positive self-evaluation;

verbalization of negative feelings about the self (helplessness, uselessness).

Minor Defining Characteristics

Self-negating verbalizations; expressions of shame/guilt; evaluates self as unable to handle situations/events; difficulty making decisions.

Related/Contributing Factors*

History of abuse (verbal, sexual, physical); chronic illness.

Sensory/Perceptual Alterations (Specify): Visual, Auditory, Kinesthetic, Gustatory, Tactile, Olfactory

A state in which an individual experiences a change in the amount or patterning of incoming stimuli accompanied by a diminished, exaggerated, distorted, or impaired response to these stimuli.

Major Defining Characteristics

Disorientation in time, place, or with persons; alteration of abstraction; altered conceptualization; change in problem-solving abilities; reported or measured change in sensory acuity; change in behavior pattern; anxiety; apathy; change in usual response to stimuli; indication of body-image alteration; restlessness; irritability; altered communication patterns.

Minor Defining Characteristics

Complaints of fatigue; alteration in posture; change in muscular tension; inappropriate responses; hallucinations.

Related Contributing Factors*

Sleep Pattern Disturbance; altered environmental stimuli, excessive or insufficient; altered sensory reception, transmission and/or integration; chemical alterations, endogenous (electrolyte), exogenous (drugs, *etc.*); psychological stress.

Sexual Dysfunction

(see also *Sexuality Patterns, Altered*)

The state in which an individual experiences a change in sexual function that is viewed as unsatisfying, unrewarding, or inadequate.

*Adapted by author.

Major Defining Characteristics

Verbalization of problem; alterations in achieving perceived sex role; actual or perceived limitation imposed by disease and/or therapy; conflicts involving values; alteration in achieving sexual satisfaction; inability to achieve desired satisfaction; seeking confirmation of desirability; alteration in relationship with significant other; change of interest in self and others.

Related/Contributing Factors

Biopsychosocial alteration of sexuality: ineffectual or absent role models; physical abuse; psychosocial abuse, (*e.g.,* harmful relationships); vulnerability; values conflict; lack of privacy; lack of significant other; altered body structure or function (pregnancy, recent childbirth, drugs, surgery, anomalies, disease process, trauma, radiation); misinformation or lack of knowledge.

Sexuality Patterns, Altered

(see also *Sexual Dysfunction*)

The state in which an individual expresses concern regarding his or her sexuality.

Major Defining Characteristics

Reported difficulties, limitations, or changes in sexual behaviors or activities.

Related/Contributing Factors

Knowledge/skill deficit about alternative responses to health-related transitions, altered body function or structure, illness or medical; lack of privacy; lack of significant other; ineffective or absent role models; conflicts with sexual orientation or variant preferences; fear of pregnancy or of acquiring a sexually transmitted disease; impaired relationship with a significant other.

Skin Integrity, Impaired

A state in which the individual's skin is altered adversely.

Major Defining Characteristics*

Disruption of skin surface; destruction of skin layers; invasion of body structures.

Related/Contributing Factors

External: hyper- or hypothermia; chemical substance; mechanical factors (shearing forces, pressure, restraint); radiation; physical immobilization; humidity.

Internal: medication; altered nutritional state (obesity, emaciation); altered metabolic state; altered circulation; altered sensation; altered pigmentation; skeletal prominence; developmental factors; immunological deficit; alterations in turgor (change in elasticity).

Skin Integrity, Potential Impaired

A state in which the individual's skin is at risk of being altered adversely.

Major Defining Characteristics/Risk Factors*

External: hypo- or hyperthermia; chemical substance; mechanical factors (shearing forces, pressure, restraint); radiation; physical immobilization; excretions/secretions; humidity.

Internal: medication; alterations in nutritional state (obesity, emaciation); altered metabolic state; altered circulation; altered sensation; altered pigmentation; skeletal prominence; developmental factors; alterations in skin turgor (change in elasticity).

Sleep Pattern Disturbance

Disruption of sleep time that causes discomfort or interferes with desired lifestyle.

Major Defining Characteristics

Verbal complaints of difficulty falling asleep; awakening earlier or later than desired; interrupted sleep; verbal complaints of not feeling well-rested; changes in behavior and performance (increasing irritability, restlessness, disorientation, lethargy, listlessness); physical signs (mild fleeting nystagmus, slight hand tremor, ptosis of eyelid, expressionless face, dark circles under eyes, frequent yawning, changes in posture); thick speech with mispronunciation and incorrect words.

Related Factors

Sensory alterations: internal (illness, psychological stress); external (environmental changes, social cues).

Social Interaction, Impaired

The state in which an individual participates in an insufficient or excessive quantity, or ineffective quality of social exchange.

Major Defining Characteristics

Verbalized or observed discomfort in social situations; verbalized or observed inability to receive or communicate a satisfying sense of belonging, caring, interest, or shared history; observed use of unsuccessful social interaction behaviors; dysfunctional interaction with peers, family and/or others.

Minor Defining Characteristic

Family report of change of style or pattern of interaction.

Related/Contributing Factors

Knowledge/skill deficit about way to enhance mutuality; communication barriers; self-concept disturbance; absence of available significant others or peers; limited physical mobility; therapeutic isolation; sociocultural dissonance; environmental barriers; altered thought processes.

Social Isolation

(see also *Communication, Impaired; Social Interaction, Impaired*)

Aloneness experienced by the individual and perceived as imposed by others and as a negative or threatened state.

Major Defining Characteristics*

Objective: absence of supportive significant other(s) (family friends, group); sad, dull affect; inappropriate or immature interests/activities for developmental age/stage; lack of communication, withdrawal, no eye contact; preoccupation with own thoughts; projection of hostility in voice, behavior; desire to be alone or exists in a subculture; evidence of physical/mental handicap or altered state of wellness; display of behavior unaccepted by dominant cultural group.

Subjective: expression of feelings of solitude imposed by others; expression of feelings of rejection; experiences of feelings different from others; inadequacy in or absence of significant purpose in life; inability to meet expectations of others; insecurity in public; expression of values acceptable to the subculture but unacceptable to the dominant cultural group; expression of interests inappropriate to the developmental age/state.

Related/Contributing Factors*

Factors contributing to the absence of satisfying personal relationships (*e.g.,* illness, lack of peers).

*Adapted by author.

Spiritual Distress

Distress of the human spirit; disruption in the life principle that pervades a person's entire being and integrates and transcends one's biological and psychosocial nature.

Major Defining Characteristics

Expresses concern with meaning of life/death and/or belief systems; anger toward God; questions about meaning of suffering; verbalization of inner conflict about beliefs; verbalization of concern about relationship with deity; questions about meaning of own existence; inability to participate in usual religious practices; search for spiritual assistance; questions about moral/ethical implications of therapeutic regimen; gallows humor; displacement of anger toward religious representatives; description of nightmares/sleep disturbances; alteration in behavior/mood evidenced by anger, crying, withdrawal, preoccupation, anxiety, hostility, apathy, *etc.*

Related/Contributing Factors

Separation from religious/cultural ties; challenged belief and value system (*e.g.,* due to moral/ethical implications of therapy or intense suffering).

Suffocating, Potential for

(see also *Home Maintenance Management, Impaired*)

The accentuated risk of accidental suffocation (inadequate air available for inhalation).

Major Defining Characteristics/Risk Factors

Individual: reduced olfactory sensation; reduced motor abilities; lack of safety education; lack of safety precautions; cognitive or emotional difficulties; disease or injury process.

Environmental: pillow placed in an infant's crib; propped bottle placed in infant's crib; vehicle warming in closed garage; children playing with plastic bags or inserting small objects into their mouths or noses; discarded or unused refrigerators or freezers without removed doors; children left unattended in bathtubs or pools; household gas leaks; smoking in bed; use of fuel-burning heaters not vented to outside; low-strung clothesline; pacifier hung around infant's head; person who eats large mouthfuls of food.

*Adapted by author.

Swallowing, Impaired

(see also *Aspiration, Potential for*)

The state in which an individual has decreased ability to voluntarily pass fluids and/or solids from the mouth to the stomach.

Major Defining Characteristic

Observed evidence of difficulty in swallowing, (*e.g.,* stasis of food in oral cavity) coughing/choking.

Minor Defining Characteristics*

Evidence of aspiration; drooling; decreased level of consciousness.

Related/Contributing Factors*

Neuromuscular impairment (*e.g.,* decreased or absent gag reflex, decreased strength or excursion of muscles involved in mastication, perceptual impairment facial paralysis); mechanical obstruction (*e.g.,* edema, tracheostomy tube, tumor); fatigue; limited awareness; reddened, irritated oropharyngeal cavity.

Thermoregulation, Ineffective

The state in which the individual's temperature fluctuates between hypothermia and hyperthermia.

Major Defining Characteristics

Fluctuations in body temperature above or below the normal range. *See also* major and minor characteristics present in *Hypothermia* and *Hyperthermia.*

Related Contributing Factors

Trauma or illness; immaturity; aging; fluctuating environmental temperature.

Thought Processes, Altered

(see also *Sensory/Perceptual Alterations*)

A state in which an individual experiences a disruption in cognitive operations and activities.

Major Defining Characteristics

Inaccurate interpretation of environment; cognitive dissonance, distractibility; memory deficit/problems; egocentricity; hyper- or hypovigilance.

Minor Defining Characteristics

Inappropriate, nonreality-based thinking.

Related/Contributing Factors*

Medications; sleep disturbance.

Tissue Integrity, Impaired

(see also *Oral Mucous Membrane, Altered; Skin Integrity, Impaired*)

Major Defining Characteristics

Damaged or destroyed tissue (cornea, mucous membrane, integumentary, or subcutaneous).

Related/Contributing Factors

Altered circulation; nutritional deficit/excess; fluid deficit/excess; knowledge deficit; impaired physical mobility; chemical irritants (including body excretions, secretions, medications); thermal irritants (temperature extremes); mechanical irritants (pressure, shear, friction); radiation (including therapeutic radiation).

Tissue Perfusion, Altered (Specify): Renal, Cerebral, Cardiopulmonary, Gastrointestinal, Peripheral

The state in which an individual experiences a decrease in nutrition and oxygenation at the cellular level because of deficit in capillary blood supply.

Major Defining Characteristics*

Decreased cardiac output; cold skin temperature; poor peripheral pulse quality blue/black pale skin; claudication; bruits, slow healing of lesions.

Related Factors*

Interruption of flow, arterial; interruption of flow, venous; exchange problems; hypovolemia; hypervolemia; organ or system pathology.

*Adapted by author.

Trauma, Potential for

(see also *Home Maintenance Management, Impaired*)

The accentuated risk of accidental tissue injury (*e.g.*, wound, burn, fracture).

Major Defining Characteristics/Risk Factors

Individual: weakness: poor vision; balancing difficulties; reduced temperature and/or tactile sensation; reduced large or small muscle coordination; reduced hand-eye coordination; lack of safety education; lack of safety precautions; insufficient finances to purchase safety equipment or effect repairs; cognitive or emotional difficulties; history of previous trauma.

Environmental: slippery floors (*e.g.*, wet or highly waxed); snow or ice collected on stairs, walkways, unanchored rugs; bathtub without hand grip or antislip equipment; use of unsteady ladders or chairs; entering unlighted rooms; unsturdy or absent stair rails; unanchored electric wires; litter or liquid spills on floors or stairways; high beds; children playing without gates at the top of the stairs; obstructed passageways; unsafe window protection in homes with young children; inappropriate call-for-aid mechanisms for bed-resting client; pot handles facing toward front of stove; bathing in very hot water (*e.g.*, unsupervised bathing of young children); potential igniting gas leaks; delayed lighting of gas burner or oven; experimenting with chemical or gasoline; unscreened fires or heaters; wearing plastic apron or flowing clothes around open flame; children playing with matches, candles, cigarettes; inadequately stored combustibles or corrosives (*e.g.*, matches, oily rags, lye); highly flammable children's toys or clothing; overloaded fuse boxes; contact with rapidly moving machinery, industrial belts, or pulleys; sliding on coarse bed linen or struggling within bed restraints; faulty electrical plugs, frayed wires, or defective appliances; contact with acids or alkalis; playing with fireworks or gunpowder; contact with intense cold; overexposure to sun, sun lamps, radiotherapy; use of cracked dishware or glasses; knives stored uncovered; guns or ammunition stored unlocked; large icicles hanging from roof; exposure to dangerous machinery; children playing with sharp-edged toys; high crime neighborhood and vulnerable clients; driving a mechanically unsafe vehicle; driving after partaking of alcoholic beverages or drugs; driving at excessive speeds; driving without necessary visual aids; children riding in the front seat of car; smoking in bed or near oxygen; overloaded electrical outlets; grease waste collected on stoves; use of thin or worn potholders or misuse of necessary headgear for motorized cyclists or young children carried on adult bicycles; unsafe road or road-crossing conditions; play or work near vehicle pathways (*e.g.*, driveways, lanes, railroad tracks); nonuse or misuse of seat restraints.

Unilateral Neglect

The state in which an individual is perceptually unaware of and inattentive to one side of the body.

Major Defining Characteristics

Consistent inattention to stimuli on an affected side.

Minor Defining Characteristics*

Inadequate self-care; inadequate positioning and/or safety precautions in regard to the affected side; does not look toward affected side; leaves food on plate on the affected side.

Related/Contributing Factors*

Effects of disturbed perceptual abilities (*e.g.,* hemianopsia; one-sided blindness; stroke; brain tumor; head injury.

Urinary Elimination, Altered Patterns of
(see also *Urinary Incontinence, Functional; Urinary Incontinence, Reflex; Urinary Incontinence, Stress; Urinary Incontinence, Total; Urinary Incontinence, Urge; and Urinary Retention*)

The state in which the individual experiences a disturbance in urine elimination.

Major Defining Characteristics

Dysuria; frequency; hesitancy; incontinence; nocturia; retention; urgency.

Related/Contributing Factors

Multiple causality, including anatomical obstruction, sensory motor impairment, urinary tract infection.

Urinary Incontinence, Functional*
(see also *Urinary Elimination, Altered Patterns of*)

The state in which an individual experiences an involuntary, unpredictable passage of urine.

Major Defining Characteristics

Urge to void or bladder contractions sufficiently strong to result in loss of urine before reaching an appropriate receptacle.

Related/Contributing Factors

Altered environment; sensory, cognitive, or mobility deficits.

Urinary Incontinence, Reflex*
(see also *Urinary Elimination, Altered Patterns of*)

The state in which an individual experiences an involuntary loss of urine, occurring at somewhat predictable intervals when a specific bladder volume is reached.

Major Defining Characteristics

No awareness of bladder filling; no urge to void or feelings of bladder fullness; uninhibited bladder contraction/spasm at regular intervals.

Related/Contributing Factors

Neurological impairment (*e.g.,* spinal cord lesion that interferes with conduction of cerebral messages above the level of the reflex arc).

Urinary Incontinence, Stress*
(see also *Urinary Elimination, Altered Patterns of*)

Major Defining Characteristics

Reported or observed dribbling with increased abdominal pressure.

Minor Defining Characteristics

Urinary urgency; urinary frequency (more often than every 2 hours).

Related/Contributing Factors

Degenerative changes in pelvic muscles and structural supports associated with increased age; high intra-abdominal pressure (*e.g.,* obesity, gravid uterus); incompetent bladder outlet; overdistention between voidings; weak pelvic muscles and structural supports.

Urinary Incontinence, Total*
(see also *Urinary Elimination, Altered Patterns of*)

The state in which an individual experiences a continuous and unpredictable loss of urine.

Major Defining Characteristics

Constant flow of urine occurs at unpredictable times without distention or uninhibited bladder contractions/spasm; unsuccessful incontinence refractory treatments; nocturia.

Minor Defining Characteristics

Lack of perineal or bladder filling awareness; unawareness of incontinence.

Related/Contributing Factors

Neuropathy preventing transmission of reflex indicating bladder fullness; neurological dysfunction causing triggering of micturition at unpredictable times; independent contraction of detrusor reflex due to surgery; trauma or disease, affecting spinal cord nerves; anomaly (fistula).

Urinary Incontinence, Urge*
(see also *Urinary Elimination, Altered Patterns of*)

The state in which an individual experiences involuntary passage of urine occurring soon after a strong sense of urgency to void.

Major Defining Characteristics

Urinary urgency; frequency (voiding more often than every two hours); bladder contracture/spasm.

Minor Defining Characteristics

Nocturia (More than two times per night); voiding in small amounts (less than 100 cc) or in large amount (more than 550 cc); inability to reach toilet in time.

Related/Contributing Factors

Decreased bladder capacity (*e.g.*, history of PID, abdominal surgeries, indwelling urinary catheter); irritation of bladder stretch receptors causing spasm (*e.g.*, bladder infection); alcohol; caffeine; increased fluids; increased urine concentration; overdistention of bladder.

Urinary Retention
(see also *Urinary Elimination, Altered Patterns of*)

The state in which the individual experiences incomplete emptying of the bladder.

Major Defining Characteristics

Bladder distention; small, frequent voiding or absence of urine output.

Minor Defining Characteristics

Sensation of bladder fullness; dribbling; residual urine; dysuria; overflow incontinence.

Related/Contributing Factors

High urethral pressure caused by weak detrusor; inhibition of reflex arc; strong sphincter; blockage.

Violence, Potential For: Self-directed or Directed at Others

A state in which an individual experiences behaviors that can be physically harmful either to the self or others.

Major Defining Characteristics

Body language (clenched fists, tense facial expression, rigid posture, tautness indicating effort to control); hostile, threatening verbalizations: boasting to or prior abuse of others; increased motor activity: pacing, excitement, irritability, agitation; overt and aggressive acts: goal-directed destruction of objects in environment; possession of destructive means: gun, knife, weapon; rage; self-destructive behavior, active aggressive suicidal acts; suspicion of others, paranoid ideation, delusions, hallucinations; substance abuse/withdrawal.

Minor Defining Characteristics

Increasing anxiety levels; fear of self or others; inability to verbalize feelings; repetition of verbalizations; continued complaints, requests, and demands; anger; provocative behavior: argumentation, dissatisfaction, overreaction, hypersensitivity; vulnerable self-esteem, depression (specifically active, aggressive, suicidal acts).

Related/Contributing Factors*

Antisocial character; history of abuse; catatonic excitement; child abuse; manic excitement; organic brain syndrome; panic states; rage reactions; suicidal behavior; temporal lobe epilepsy; toxic reactions to medication.

Appendices

Appendix A. Requirements for Submitting a Proposed New Nursing Diagnosis*

Components

A. *Name:* This part provides a name for diagnosis, a concise phrase, term, or label.

B. *Definition:* This part provides a clear, precise definition of the named diagnosis. The definition expresses the essential nature of the diagnosis named and delineates its meaning. The definition should enable one to differentiate this diagnosis from all others.

C. *Defining Characteristics:* This part provides a list of observable cues that the client presents that substantiate for the nurse that the nursing judgment (*e.g.*, the selected diagnosis) appropriately labels and describes the client state, the phenomena of concern. Cues must be both listed and defined. Cues are separated into two positions or sets: major and minor.

  1. *Major Defining Characteristics:* Those that appear to be present in all clients experiencing the phenomena of concern.

  2. *Minor Defining Characteristics:* Those that appear to be present in many clients experiencing the phenomena of concern.

D. *Substantiating/Supportive Materials:* This part provides documentation that substantiates the existence, nature, and characteristics of the phenomena of concern. Minimal validation documentation is a listing of references demonstrating a reasonable review of relevant literature. Narrative materials accompanying such a reference list may not exceed 1500 words.

Optional Components for Submission of a Proposed New Nursing Diagnosis

A. *Supplemental Information:* The following types of supplemental information may be submitted to further clarify the nursing phenomena identified by the proposed nursing diagnosis.

  1. *Related Factors:** In some cases, there may be specific factors that appear to show some type of patterned relationship with the phenomena of concern, named as a nursing diagnosis. Where this situation exists, it may be helpful to name and describe these. Such factors may be described variously as antecedent to, associated with, related to, contributing to, or abetting.

(Reprinted with permission from the North American Nursing Diagnosis Association. Submissions should be mailed to NANDA, University School of Nursing, 3525 Caroline Street, St. Louis, MO 63104)

*Etiology was deleted as a requirement for submission but can be optional.

2. *Sources of Variance:* In some cases, unique sources of variance in the experience of the phenomena may be possible. Where this situation exists, it may be helpful to identify these. Such sources of variance may include developmental stage variance, ethnic or cultural variance, levels of risk variance, acuity variance, and multi-diagnosis variance.

B. *Supplemental Validation:* If it is available, supplemental validation of the nursing diagnosis may be submitted. This may include research abstracts, brief reports of validation projects, or reports of intervention or treatment studies. These must be brief in character, not exceeding 1500 words.

Appendix B. North American Nursing Diagnosis Association Diagnosis Review Cycle

The North American Nursing Diagnosis Association (NANDA), in an effort to meet its purpose "to develop, refine, and promote a taxonomy of nursing diagnostic terminology of general use to professional nurses," has developed a formal cycle of diagnosis review to enable the process of incorporation of new diagnoses submitted by interested parties. This process is cyclic in character, assuring continuous development and refinement of the taxonomy.

Step 1. Receipt of Diagnoses: Diagnoses may be entered into the review cycle either on the initiative of NANDA or others.

A. NANDA initiates this process by soliciting diagnoses, advertising of their interest in diagnoses, publishing their guidelines for submission, and responding to inquiries concerning such guidelines.

B. Individual nurses or nurse groups initiate this process by submitting a diagnosis for review. When a submission is received by NANDA, it is initially reviewed for compliance with submission guidelines. Those submissions that involve only a suggested name or are only partially developed are returned to the person submitting the recommendation with a request for completion as described in the guidelines. Those submissions that meet criteria of the guidelines then enter the review process. The person submitting the suggested diagnosis receives a copy of the description of the Diagnosis Review Cycle at this time, to facilitate an understanding of NANDA's policies and procedures.

Step 2. Diagnoses Enter the Public Domain: NANDA formally recognizes all diagnoses under review as part of the public domain. As such, any diagnosis submitted for review is briefly reported in the *NANDA Newsletter* when it enters the review cycle. Persons submitting diagnoses are advised of this fact and are asked to indicate in writing their acceptance of this policy on a form provided by NANDA.

It is recognized, however, that individuals have often invested considerable time and energy in an effort to delineate one or more diagnoses. Therefore, the publication of a diagnoses entering the review cycle will include the name of the person(s) submitting this diagnosis, assuring them of recognition of their efforts. This will also improve networking and communication among members actively engaged in exploring common or comparable diagnoses.

Step 3. Diagnoses Are Reviewed by Clinical Technical Task Forces: The NANDA Diagnosis Review Committee (DRC) is charged with the task of reviewing proposed diagnoses and recommending their acceptance, modification, or rejection to the NANDA Board. This committee's work is guided by the advice and critique of clinical/technical task forces who review diagnoses.

A. Each diagnosis accepted for review is assigned by the Chairperson of the Diagnosis Review Committee (DRC) to a member of that committee. This person serves as a primary or lead reviewer of the diagnosis and the Chairperson of the Clinical/Technical Review Task Force, which will review the diagnosis.

B. The Clinical/Technical Review Task Force is a panel created to review a specific diagnosis based on individual clinical and technical expertise. Task force members are drawn not only from NANDA membership, but also from expert groups in organizations such as the Canadian Nurses' Association and the American Nurses' Association. NANDA board members who do not serve on the Diagnosis Review Committee (DRC) are ineligible to serve on these task forces. Task forces are created as needed and appropriate by the Diagnosis Review Committee (DRC).

C. Members of the various task forces receive diagnoses for critique and review with an evaluation form provided. This evaluation form enables reviewers to assess the degree to which the diagnosis submitted meets the criteria of the submission guidelines. Task force members are given two to four weeks to respond to a request for a review. These reviews are forwarded to the primary reviewer.

D. Based on task force members' advice and comments, the primary reviewer prepares a diagnosis proposal for each diagnosis. These are presented at a meeting of the Diagnosis Review Committee.

Step 4. Diagnoses Are Reviewed by the NANDA Diagnosis Review Committee: The Diagnosis Review Committee convenes to review, discuss, and take action on the proposals for new diagnoses prepared by the primary reviewers of the Clinical/Technical Task Forces. Three possible outcomes emerge from this process.

A. The DRC accepts the proposed diagnosis or makes minor changes, or

B. The DRC substantively alters the diagnosis as submitted by the original proposer, based on reviewer advice. The DRC then accepts the proposed diagnosis, or

C. The DRC rejects the diagnosis and identifies specific reasons for the rejection. In this case, the original proposer of the diagnosis is provided with specific recommendations for improvement.

The DRC notifies the original proposer of the diagnosis of their action at this time. They concurrently forward their recommendations to the NANDA Board.

Step 5. Diagnoses Are Reviewed by the NANDA Board: The NANDA Board receives the recommendations of the DRC and convenes to review, discuss, and take action on the DRC recommendations. Once more, three possible outcomes emerge from this process.

A. The Board accepts the DRC recommendation, or

B. The Board returns the diagnosis to the DRC with comments for revision and recommendations for change, or

C. The Board rejects the DRC recommendation and identifies specific reasons for the rejection.

The DRC then notifies the original proposer of the Board's action and prepares accepted diagnoses for General Assembly review and comment.

Step 6. Diagnoses Are Reviewed by the General Assembly: The General Assembly has the authority to review and comment on proposed diagnoses for the DRC's actions prior to the submission to the membership for acceptance. The DRC prepares proposed diagnoses for this review and comment. The DRC therefore engages in the following activities:

A. The DRC groups the diagnoses as possible or appropriate for General Assembly review.

B. The DRC structures time for review and comment by the General Assembly during the National Conference, advising the original proposer of the diagnosis of this action.

C. The DRC develops policies, procedures, and protocols for General Assembly review and comment and conducts these sessions accordingly.

D. The DRC collects General Assembly comments and incorporates these into proposed diagnoses as appropriate and feasible.

E. The DRC reports these changes to the Board.

Step 7. Diagnoses Are Voted Upon by the NANDA Membership: The DRC prepares diagnoses for a NANDA membership vote. This includes several activities.

A. The DRC creates a mail ballot of proposed diagnoses to be distributed to all current NANDA members.

B. The DRC oversees the distribution and tallying of ballots. They record any suggestions for needed subsequent revision of any given diagnosis.

C. The DRC communicates information on the outcome of balloting to the original proposer of the diagnoses. Unapproved diagnoses can be revised and can reenter the cycle. Approved diagnoses become a part of the approved NANDA Taxonomy.

D. The DRC forwards the approved diagnoses to the National Conference Proceedings editor for inclusion in the Proceedings and to the Taxonomy Committee for inclusion in the NANDA Taxonomy.

(Reprinted with permission from the North American Nursing Diagnosis Association. Submissions should be mailed to NANDA, University School of Nursing, 3525 Caroline Street, St. Louis, MO 63104)

Appendix C. NANDA Diagnosis Qualifiers

Category 1

Actual: Existing at the present moment; existing in reality

Potential: Can, but has not yet, come into being; possible

Category 2

Ineffective: Not producing the desired effect; not capable of performing satisfactorily

Decreased: Smaller; lessened; diminished; lesser in size, amount, or degree

Increased: Greater in size, amount or degree; larger, enlarged

Impaired: Made worse, weakened; damaged, reduced; deteriorated

Depleted: Emptied wholly or partially; exhausted of

Deficient: Inadequate in amount, quality, or degree; defective; not sufficient; incomplete

Excessive: Characterized by an amount or quantity that is greater than necessary, desirable, or usable

Dysfunctional: Abnormal; impaired or incompletely functioning

Disturbed: Agitated; interrupted, interfered with

Acute: Severe but of short duration

Chronic: Lasting a long time; recurring; habitual; constant

Intermittent: Stopping and starting again at intervals; periodic; cyclic

(Reprinted with permission from the North American Nursing Diagnosis Association, St. Louis, MO, 1986)

Index

A

Abdominal surgery, standard of nursing care, 97
Activity intolerance, 184
  potential, 184
Adjustment, impaired, 184
Affective domain (client outcome), 105
Airway clearance, ineffective, 184
American Nurses' Association (ANA)
  Social Policy Statement (1980), 55
  Standards of Nursing Practice, 96. *See also Standards of Nursing Practice*
Anxiety, 184–185
Aspiration, potential for, 185
Assessment, 3, 13–50
  authority to perform, 58
  communicating/recording data, 48–49
  components of, 14–15
  data base, 14
  data collection, 15–39
  data organization (clustering), 41–47
  data validation, 39–41
  definition, 2
  in evaluating client goal achievement, 157
  focus. *See* Focus assessment
  glossary of terms, 14
  key points, 49–50
  as nursing intervention, 108
  pattern identification and filling in gaps, 47–48
  physical, 32–35
  relation to diagnosis, 4–6
Audit, 156
Auscultation, 32

B

Baseline data, 14
Body image disturbance, 185
Body systems, data organization according to, 42, 45
Body temperature, potential altered, 185
Bowel incontinence, 185
Breastfeeding, ineffective, 186
Breathing pattern, ineffective, 186

C

V

Validation
   of assessment data, 39–41
   definition, 14
   of nursing diagnosis, PES format for, 70–72
Variables, 156
   goal achievement and, 159–160
Verbal communication, 48, 150–152
   change-of-shift report, 150–152
Verbs
   measurable, 90, 101
   nonmeasurable, 101
   representative of affective, cognitive and psychomotor domains, 105
Violence, potential for: self-directed or directed at others, 206

W

Wellness, definition, 55